How to develop

numeracy

in children with dyslexia

Pauline Clayton

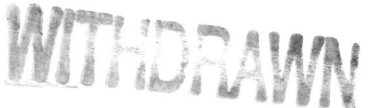
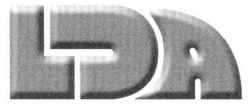

Acknowledgements

This book would not have been written without the following individuals, to whom I am indebted.

Firstly, Margaret Rooms of Dyslexia Action.

Secondly, colleagues within Dyslexia Action.

Thirdly, experienced and well-known experts in the field of dyslexia and mathematics – particularly Dr S. Chinn (Mark College, Somerset) and also Professor M. Sharma (Institute of Mathematics, Massachusetts), whose philosophies have formed the basis of many of the teaching ideas I now use.

Fourthly, the learners I have taught who have, in return, taught me a great deal about maths and dyslexia.

Fifthly, the staff at LDA for producing this book from my initial manuscript.

Lastly, my husband, who has tolerated the stress.

Permission to photocopy

This book contains materials which may be reproduced by photocopier or other means for use by the purchaser. The permission is granted on the understanding that these copies will be used within the educational establishment of the purchaser. The book and all its contents remain copyright. Copies may be made without reference to the publisher or the licensing scheme for the making of photocopies operated by the Publishers' Licensing Agency.

The right of Pauline Clayton to be identified as the author of this work has been asserted by her in accordance with sections 77 and 78 of the Copyright, Designs and Patents Act 1988.

How to develop numeracy in children with dyslexia
MT00600
ISBN-13: 978 1 85503 379 5
© Pauline Clayton
Cover illustration © Peter Wilks
Inside illustrations © Rebecca Barnes
All rights reserved
First published 2003
Reprinted 2004 (March, August), 2005, 2007, 2008 (twice)

Printed in the UK for LDA
Abbeygate House, East Road, Cambridge, CB1 1DB, UK

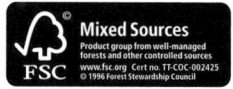

Contents

Contents

Introduction   4

1   *Chapter 1*   5
The connections

2   *Chapter 2*   12
Testing and assessment

3   *Chapter 3*   20
Dyslexia and the Primary Framework for mathematics

4   *Chapter 4*   26
Focus on mathematics

5   *Chapter 5*   35
Strategies for support

6   *Chapter 6*   49
Making maths multi-sensory

7   *Chapter 7*   53
Final thoughts

Photocopiable resources   54
Resources   63

Introduction

This book takes the difficulties encountered by pupils with dyslexia into the mathematical environment. In my time as a teacher I have worked with many individuals with dyslexia, both children and adults, who have also encountered problems with maths or, more often, numeracy in general. I have become increasingly aware, as have many other teachers and also parents, that some dyslexic children experience difficulties in mathematics.

There are a number of children who do not have any difficulty in literacy but do have a specific difficulty in maths. These children are sometimes called *dyscalculic* (unable to calculate). Present research indicates that they benefit from teaching that follows the same principles as those recommended when working with children with dyslexia.

Many books have been written to support the teaching of mathematics in accordance with national guidelines and this book does not attempt to echo those. The areas of particular concern are considered and suggestions made.

The book will help you to:

◑ gain an understanding of the links between dyslexia and maths;

◑ look at the Primary National Strategy (PNS) in relation to dyslexia;

◑ look at the skills necessary for children with dyslexia to succeed at maths;

◑ explore some ideas to support children with dyslexia in the mathematics classroom.

The philosophy throughout this book can be summed up as follows:

Make maths multi-sensory.

Interest in the relationship between dyslexia and maths is growing rapidly, as more teachers and parents become aware of children's difficulties. This book will be one more step along the way towards the understanding, teaching and support of our pupils with dyslexia in the mathematics classroom.

Chapter 1
The connections

This chapter covers the following areas:

- Definitions of dyslexia and mathematics used in this book.
- Problems a dyslexic individual may experience in the learning environment.
- An introduction to dyscalculia.
- Arithmetic and numeracy.
- Skills needed to master mathematics.
- Specific problem areas.
- The difference between numeracy and mathematics.

Before discussing dyslexia and mathematics certain definitions must be agreed.

Dyslexia

The definition used here is that of Dyslexia Action (2007):

> Dyslexia is a specific learning difficulty that mainly affects reading and spelling. It is characterised by difficulties in processing word-sounds and by weaknesses in short-term verbal memory; its effects may be seen in both written and spoken language. The current evidence suggests that these difficulties arise from inefficiencies in language-processing areas in the left hemisphere of the brain which, in turn, appear to be linked to genetic differences.
>
> Dyslexia is not related to intelligence, race or social background. Its effects can be minimised by targeted literacy intervention, technological support and adaptations to ways of working and learning.

Areas of possible difficulty

See the chart on page 6. For further information see Neanon (2002).

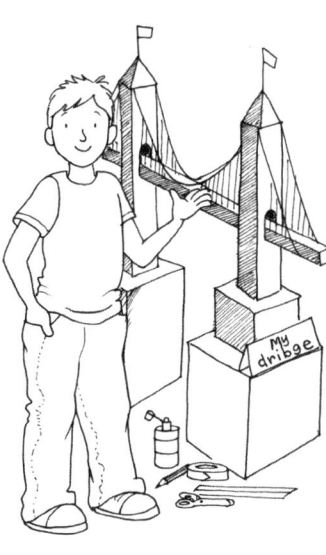

Dyslexia is generally understood to relate to literacy and language, but many parents, teachers and researchers are aware that it may also relate to mathematics. Not all children with dyslexic problems will experience difficulties in mathematics. Some make good mathematicians; others show strengths in the more practical mathematics-related subjects such as physics, engineering and architecture. Little research has been done to assess the percentage of children with dyslexia experiencing difficulties with mathematics. However, Joffe (1981) suggests that 60 per cent of dyslexic individuals have problems severe enough to require remediation. Miles and Miles (1991) see this figure as simplistic: 'It may be that all dyslexics have some difficulties with mathematics (as part and parcel of their problems with language and memory) but there is considerable variation in the extent to which these difficulties are overcome.'

Areas of possible difficulty

A dyslexic individual may experience difficulties in any of the following areas.

Reading	decoding, understanding, comprehension, fluency
Memory	short-term and working memory, moving information into long-term memory; recalling that information
Handwriting	this may be poorly formed and letters/symbols may be incorrectly written
Spelling	phoneme recognition, transferring phonemes to the correct grapheme, visual recognition of correct/incorrect spelling
Sequencing and logical thinking	problems may occur in: writing letters in words or digits in numbers in the correct order, correctly sequencing procedures, problem solving
Visual perception and processing	problems with: keeping place when reading, reading letters/words/symbols, interpreting diagrams correctly
Speed of information processing	information is processed more slowly so work often progresses too fast in the classroom, meaning that the learner does not have sufficient practice to master concepts and procedures
Concentration	the brain of a child with dyslexia is 'wired differently' and the learner has to work harder to achieve the same standard as their peers; this means that their level of concentration cannot be retained for as long as may be required for learning in the classroom
Organisation	poor organisational skills affect many areas – from taking the right books to school to organising project work
Time management	it is widely recognised that many children with dyslexia have difficulty in telling the time, but what may be less well understood is that they may also have difficulty in recognising the passage of time; this particularly affects project work and examinations
Confidence and self-esteem	low confidence and self-esteem mean that, apart from having a poor self-image, learners are reluctant to participate in learning; the learners themselves are the best predictors of their levels of performance, thus a learner with low confidence levels will achieve work at a lower level than they are capable of, given suitable support

Dyscalculia

Teachers, parents and psychologists are becoming increasingly aware of children who, although not dyslexic, are having specific difficulties with mathematics. These children are often called dyscalculic. Dyscalculia is gaining recognition as a specific learning difficulty.

> Dyscalculia is a developmental, or acquired, disorder that results in an inability to do or to learn mathematics, particularly arithmetic. This means difficulties in some or all of the following: mastering simple number concepts, understanding number relationships, understanding spatial relationships, and learning algorithms and applying them. It is most commonly revealed through substantially lowered arithmetical achievement, sometimes several years below the appropriate level.

A large number of dyslexic individuals will have difficulties in some or all areas of mathematics. Dyscalculia can exist alone; it need not be accompanied by any difficulty in literacy.

At present, knowledge, research and understanding of dyscalculia lag well behind that of dyslexia. The present recommendation is that these children should be taught using the principles that are recommended for the teaching of pupils with dyslexia – structured, cumulative and multi-sensory.

Thus, whether addressing the needs of the dyslexic or the dyscalculic learner, we need to make maths multi-sensory, which is the theme of this book.

Mathematics

To link dyslexia with mathematics we must also have a clear definition of mathematics, such as the following one.

> Mathematics is a symbolic language used to: express relationships – spatial, numerical, geometric, algebraic and trigonometric, in both real and imaginary dimensions; communicate concepts through symbols; reinforce and practise sequential and logical thinking.

Whilst looking at definitions, it is also worth defining both arithmetic and numeracy.

> Arithmetic is the branch of mathematics concerned with numerical calculations, such as addition, subtraction, multiplication and division.
>
> Numeracy has been described as literacy with numbers. It is the recognition of numbers and operators, and the appreciation of how these can be combined to form arithmetical problems.

It can be argued that the term 'numeracy' means the same as 'arithmetic' but the former has, to a large extent, superseded the latter. In this book I shall use the term 'numeracy' for ease of reference.

Numeracy and mathematics

It is also important to be aware of the difference between numeracy and mathematics. Some examples should make this clear.

- ◑ A physics graduate who still has trouble with the 7-times table has a numeracy problem.
- ◑ A pupil who cannot generalise numerical patterns has mathematical problems.

Numeracy is part of maths – a large part at primary level, but smaller at secondary level and beyond.

Much of numeracy – or arithmetic – is taught by repetition and practice. That is fine, except that, as previously pointed out, many pupils with dyslexia are slower than others at reading, understanding and processing information – that is working out what they have to do, and actually doing it. This often means that, for example, when presented with ten questions and a limited time the dyslexic child may only answer five. These answers may be correct but the child does not gain as much practice as their non-dyslexic peers and is therefore less likely to remember what has been learned.

If the speed of information processing reduces the amount of reinforcement at every stage of mathematics, then the learning of each stage will be incomplete.

The main skills needed to learn mathematics

If we accept that a certain level of general cognitive ability is needed by all learners studying mathematics, we then need to look at the main skills needed to learn the subject and consider what can happen if you are dyslexic.

Before you read further, try to complete the table supplied (see page 9). Now look at the completed table (pages 10–11) to compare your responses.

Conclusion

We need clear definitions of the terms we use. We must also realise that not every child with dyslexia will display all of the above weaknesses and difficulties. In fact, a high proportion of learners will show strengths in certain areas, especially in spatial skills. The greater the number of specific problem areas that are experienced by a child, the greater the effect on the child's learning and understanding of mathematics.

Having looked at the terminology that covers the area of numeracy and dyslexia, we turn in Chapter 2 to the ways in which we can identify a child with dyslexia who may be having difficulties with numeracy.

'Many pupils with dyslexia are slower than others at reading, understanding and processing information.'

The main skills needed to learn mathematics

Mathematical skill	How it relates to maths	What may happen if you are dyslexic
Ability to visualise		
Perception skills		
Processing skills		
Language ability		
Spatial ability		
Sequential thinking		
Logical thinking		
Linking		
Estimation		
Memory		
Confidence and self-esteem		

The main skills needed in mathematics

Completed table

Mathematical skill	How it relates to maths	What may happen if you are dyslexic
Ability to visualise	Picturing questions in your head. Seeing geometrical shapes, how numbers are written, how they relate to each other.	This may be a strength. If not, then the problems are in linking two-dimensional drawings to their three-dimensional originals, and in seeing numbers as symbols that bear no relationship to each other, or to the real world.
Perception skills	Interpreting diagrams, reading digits and numbers, understanding relationships. Choosing the correct method or formula to solve a question.	Not understanding a relationship or diagram in the same way as the teacher does will make learning difficult or even impossible.
Processing skills	The speed and efficiency with which information is taken in, manipulated and given out.	Often slow, so less practice and reinforcement result. Because of poor memory skills, more reinforcement is what is needed.
Language ability	Reading (decoding) a question, both words and symbols; understanding what has been read in a mathematical sense.	Poor language skills hinder decoding and also the understanding of many English words used in a mathematical context.
Spatial ability	Linked to visualisation. Relating shapes, objects, digits, numbers, symbols to each other and recognising patterns. At an early stage, understanding that the number of objects is unaffected by the space they take up.	Often a strength; however, those learners with poor spatial skills may write numbers and symbols incorrectly, rely on rote learning and – although able to 'do' some numeracy – experience difficulty in other areas of maths.
Sequential thinking	Counting, seeing patterns in numbers and symbols. Following correct procedures to solve a questions, e.g. multiplication of 2-digit numbers by 2-digit numbers.	Poor mastery of procedures and standard methods of recording. Lack of recognition of patterns and relationships.
Logical thinking	Overlaps with the above, but involves thinking in the correct order for problem solving. Recognising patterns.	Inability to think through a problem in a correct, logical order. Failure to establish and recognise patterns.

The main skills needed in mathematics

Completed table continued

Mathematical skill	How it relates to maths	What may happen if you are dyslexic
Linking	Affected by processing speed and memory. Naming numbers and symbols. Knowing names of shapes, number bonds, multiplication tables.	Poor mastery of language of maths, relating names to shapes and symbols. Poor recall of names for shapes and vice versa.
Estimation	Ability to see the size of an answer without having to work it out exactly.	Develops with exposure to many similar examples. As children with dyslexia often get less practice, they see fewer examples to help them to improve estimation skills.
Memory	Remembering questions and instructions, following procedures. Learning number bonds, multiplication tables, new information. Solving mental calculations, recalling information from long-term memory.	Weakness in all of these areas.
Confidence and self-esteem	Willingness to tackle questions for which the solution is not immediately clear.	Lack of confidence and self-esteem means that learners are reluctant to tackle any question which stretches them.

Chapter 2
Testing and assessment

This chapter looks at:

○ warning signs that teachers, teaching assistants and parents may notice indicating possible difficulties in mathematics;

○ testing and assessment.

Warning signs for parents and teachers

Teachers often know intuitively when a pupil has a problem in maths that is not solely one of low ability across the board. There are also specific signs to look for. The child with dyslexia often shows an imbalance of skills.

The pointers in the chart on page 13 are probably relevant to learners aged 8+. Pointers vary according to the age and ability of the child. Don't forget that we can all suddenly fail to recall an addition or multiplication fact, especially if put on the spot. This does not mean we are all dyslexic; rather that we are all human.

The child who persistently has difficulties in a majority of the areas in the chart should be at least supported within the classroom and at best given an assessment to attempt to quantify their difficulty.

Assessment

Whilst there are several tests available for teachers to use with learners when dyslexia is suspected, these tests are language based and will not highlight difficulties in mathematics. Chinn (2000) has devised an individual diagnostic test to highlight areas of difficulty. Butterworth (2003) has devised a test for dyscalculia for learners aged 6–14.

There are, of course, numeracy tests available. It is not sufficient to test solely for mathematical attainment. Doing that will not show how a child's dyslexic problems affect their performance in mathematics. Rather, we must think about:

○ innate ability;

○ attainment;

○ diagnosing areas of difficulty.

The diagram on page 14 shows how these three areas of assessment are linked. It shows some of the specific tests that may be used for assessment. See the charts on pages 15–17 for information about these. We need to look for any inconsistencies in the test results. For example, a learner with a specific problem will have a mismatch of scores, whereas a learner of lower ability will probably score at a similar level on all tests and their results will reflect their

'The child with dyslexia often shows an imbalance of skills.'

Pointers

Telling the time	Is the child having difficulty learning to tell the time from an analogue clock?
Days of the week and months of the year	Is the child having difficulty remembering the days of the week and months of the year in order?
Writing numbers	Do they persist in writing digits the wrong way round? Do they reverse teen numbers, for example writing 16 as 61?
Counting backwards or in multiples	Do they find it difficult to count backwards from 20? Do they find it difficult to count in 2s, 5s and 3s etc.?
Reading numbers and operators (+, -, x, ÷, =)	Do they confuse 2 and 5, 6 and 9, + and x or + and ÷?
Visual puzzles	Do they find jigsaws and other visual puzzles difficult?
Reading and understanding words in a mathematical context	Can they read a question? Do they understand what they have read?
Mental calculation	Do they find it hard to work in their head? Is their work better if written down?
Learning number bonds	Are they finding it difficult to learn addition and subtraction facts? If older, are they having difficulty learning multiplication facts?
Addition and subtraction	Do they use fingers to count on to add? Do they always start at 1 to add two numbers?
Following correct methods and procedures	Do they find it difficult to follow a correct method to complete a calculation successfully?
Working in class and homework	Do they often not finish set tasks? Do they consistently spend longer on homework than the school has suggested?
Anxiety and confidence	Are they anxious about maths lessons? Are they reluctant to tackle questions set in class or for homework?

ability. Comparing ability and attainment allows us, as teachers, to have a realistic idea of what the learner can achieve. Diagnosing the specific mathematical areas that cause the most difficulty allows us to write a realistic Individual Education Plan (IEP) with relevant targets.

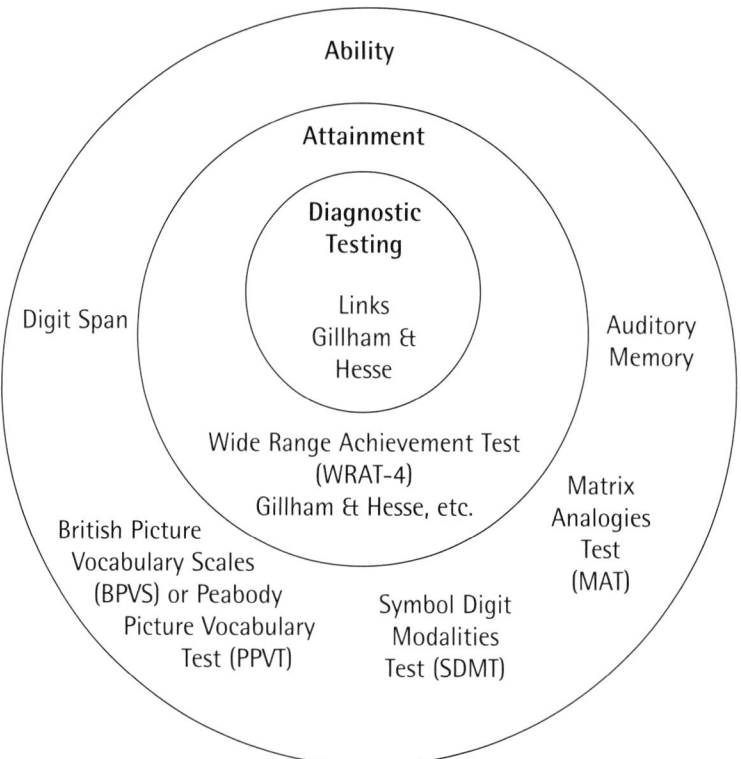

Procedure

In an ideal world, many of us would like a child to have had a full assessment by an educational psychologist prior to any assessment undertaken by a teacher. The psychologist's report should indicate the child's strengths and weaknesses. Although the main area of concern is often that of literacy, all reports will contain, either explicitly or implicitly, information on performance relating to mathematics.

At present some local education authorities (LEAs) are replacing formal assessments with less formal observational assessments carried out by class teachers. This procedure of assessing needs is regarded as 'graduated'. It recognises that children learn and develop at different rates. The starting point is teachers, parents and teaching assistants becoming aware that a problem or weakness is being experienced by a child in the school environment. The Special Educational Needs Coordinator (SENCo) has responsibility for children with special needs within the school. Discussion should follow between the teacher or SENCo, and the parent. This may lead to outside specialists being consulted.

The initial two levels of help are known as School Action and School Action Plus. It is hoped that the needs of most pupils can be met within the classroom (School Action), sometimes with the help of outside specialists (School Action Plus).

'The starting point is teachers, parents and teaching assistants becoming aware that a problem or weakness is being experienced by a child in the school environment.'

For a few pupils with more serious needs the LEA can make an assessment; if the LEA decides that special help is needed beyond that already being given, they must draw up a statement of special educational needs for the child. Parents can also ask for an assessment. How the assessment is conducted – whether it is a formal assessment or a less formal observational assessment – is not laid down.

Until very recently difficulties in maths were not recognised to the same extent as those in literacy. Greater awareness of pupils who experience problems in maths should mean that any method of assessment, whether formal or informal, can be geared more to the area of maths, if that is the main concern, or to maths and literacy if there is a problem with both.

There is a record sheet in the photocopiable resources designed specifically for use in the mathematics classroom.

For children who have had no previous assessment there are tests available to teachers, SENCos and teaching assistants to enable you to look at the three areas of ability, attainment and diagnosis, so that you can begin the process of diagnosis in school.

Ability tests

Name of test	Aim	Age range	Time to administer	Method of delivery	Supplier
Either: British Picture Vocabulary Scales (BPVS) or: Peabody Picture Vocabulary Test (PPVT)	Tests receptive vocabulary	3–15 years $2\frac{1}{2}$–adult	5–8 minutes 5–8 minutes	For both tests, the individual is presented with a set of 4 pictures and told a single word. They then have to point to, or give the number of, the picture that relates to that word.	nferNelson Dyslexia Action
Matrix Analogies Test (MAT), short form	Tests non-verbal ability and includes: pattern completion, reasoning by analogy, serial reasoning, spatial visualisation. This tests short-term/ working memory	From 5 up to 18 years	Time limit of 25 minutes	The child is led through an example and then works independently through the test.	Harcourt Assessment

Ability tests continued

A digit span test		5–adult	2–5 minutes	The individual is given an increasing number of digits, at 1-second intervals, and asked to repeat them in the correct order. They are then given further sets and asked to repeat them, but in the reverse order to that given.	Part of the Dyslexia Screening Test (DST) from Harcourt Assessment
Symbol Digit Modalities Test (SDMT)	Similar to the coding test on the Weschler Intelligence Scale (WISC). The test measures: concentration, facility with printed symbols, rapid decision making, visual–motor speed	8–adult	90 seconds	Individuals are asked to write single digits to correspond with a variety of symbols, as shown in a model.	Dyslexia Action

Additional test
The One-minute Number Test©
This normed test by Westwood *et al.* (1974) not only tests knowledge of very basic number bonds, but also speed of recalling information. Some dyslexic pupils show a marked discrepancy between the addition and the subtraction scores. (A normed test is one that has been given to a large number of individuals. The results are used to compile a table showing the scores obtained for a variety of ages. The performance of other individuals can be measured against these scores.)

Attainment tests
There is a wide variety of tests which can be used for attainment. The chart on page 17 lists some of these.

Name of test	Aim	Age range	Time to administer	Method of delivery	Supplier
Gillham & Hesse Basic Number Screening Test	To assess competence in basic number skills	7–12 years	Untimed, but approx. 20 minutes individually, up to 35 minutes for group administration	No language on test paper; instructions given by teacher, two practice items	Hodder & Stoughton
Wide Range Achievement Test (WRAT-4)	To assess arithmetical and algebraic skills (limited reading required)*	5–95 years	15 minutes for age 8+; extra oral section for younger children	Group or individual; worked through independently by individuals	Dyslexia Action
6–14 Tests of Mathematical Attainment	Designed particularly for classroom use; assesses mathematical skills (reading involved at all but lowest levels)	6–14 years	45 minutes upwards, depending on level of test used	Group or individual; early test administered orally	nferNelson

* Although this test covers a very wide age range, its advantage is that the results for the reading, spelling and maths are normed from the same extensive population. The tests should give good comparisons in performance between these three skills.

Diagnostic assessment

Diagnostic assessment involves finding out how the learner is thinking, how they are interpreting questions and mathematical symbols, and whether they can access language. Two possible tests are suggested below.

Name of test	Aim	Age range	Time to administer	Method of delivery	Supplier
Gillham & Hesse Basic Number Screening Test	To assess competence in basic number skills	7–12 years	Untimed, but approx. 20 minutes individually, up to 35 minutes for group administration	No language on test paper; instructions given by teacher, two practice items	Hodder & Stoughton
Maths Links Tests of Mastery	To link every question to a specific area of mathematics; solely a diagnostic test	Level 1 7–9 years; Level 2 10–12 years and low-attaining older pupils	Untimed; minimum 15 minutes	Level 1 – oral instructions; Level 2 – written instructions given on test paper	NASEN

'It is important that you gain an awareness of the child's innate ability as well as their attainment.'

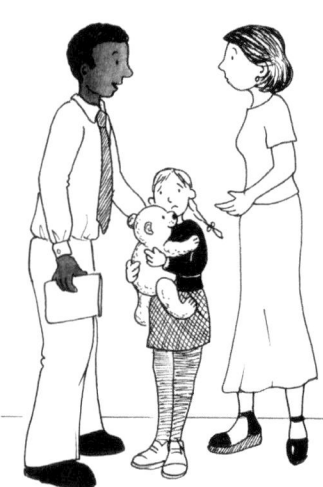

"Beth seems a little anxious about numeracy."

To gain the most information from any diagnostic test it is important to work through it with the child. This does not mean teaching and helping mathematically; it means gathering further information by:

○ talking to the child;

○ offering different language and symbols if the first presentation is not understood;

○ asking how a question was done;

○ finding out why a question cannot be answered;

○ keeping notes about the child's methods, use of language and general responses.

Many other tests are available and, providing the level of the test is suitable for the pupil, can be used successfully.

Following the introduction of the National Numeracy Strategy (NNS) the format of some older or American tests for ability and attainment may not be recognised by younger pupils. This will affect their ability to answer questions. The way a test is presented, interpreted and understood will affect the individual's ability to achieve success. Normed tests have been designed and tested in a standard format and they should probably not be rewritten; that may affect the scoring. However, when using a diagnostic test an alternative presentation can be used. This may well add to the information gained about an individual's performance.

For a diagnostic test the method of administration is more important than the actual test chosen.

The use of a calculator is not allowed in a diagnostic test situation. However, for older pupils it may be worth asking them to attempt a test twice (WRAT-4 and Gillham & Hesse have two alternative parallel tests), the second time getting them to use a different-coloured pen and a calculator. This will show how much reliance there is on a calculator, how efficient the pupil is at using one, and the extent, if any, to which estimates and checks are undertaken to ensure the correct answer.

It is not sufficient to ask the pupil to complete only the mathematical elements of a diagnostic test. It is important that you gain an awareness of the child's innate ability as well as their attainment. As discussed earlier in this chapter, comparing ability and attainment allows us, as teachers, to get a realistic idea of what the learner can achieve. A high-ability individual can be expected to achieve above their chronological age, whereas a low-ability individual can be expected to achieve below their chronological age. We must set realistic targets, ones related to ability rather than to chronological age.

Diagnostic testing takes time but it is necessary to develop a teaching programme relevant to the learner. Each of us is an individual. Effective differentiation in the classroom, and support offered, must draw on the child's strengths whilst supporting their weaknesses. Pupils with dyslexia, especially those with strengths in mathematics, often develop strategies that may seem alien to those we, as teachers, would use. We should not dismiss these. If they are mathematically sound, we can in fact often build on them.

For example, I worked with a Year-6 pupil, Sean, who understood the majority of mathematical concepts. He had a major problem with sequencing and found that, whilst he could subtract using a variety of mental strategies, when faced with a standard written method, he became very muddled. He devised a way of transferring what he was doing mentally onto paper. I have attempted to show his logic here.

Example

642	*Sean's thinking*		*Notes*
- 258			
		642	First he subtracted the hundreds,
		- 258	then the tens, then the units.
	Start on the left and take 2 from 6.	442	Here he omitted the 2 (hundred)
	I can't take 5 from 4 so I need the 44. To	- 58	Here he omitted the 5 (tens)
	take 5 from 44 I can take 10 and add 5.	392	
	This means 44 - 10 is 34. 34 + 5 is 39	- 8	
		384	
	I can't take 8 from 2 so I need the 92.		
	To take 8 I can take 10 and add 2. So		
	92 - 10 is 82 and 82 + 2 is 84		

I found this method difficult to follow, but it is mathematically sound and Sean and I were happy to work with it.

By way of a contrast, I remember Robert, a teenager, who told me with glee that he had mastered percentages. His logic was simple. He had realised that to find 10 per cent of a number he could divide the number by 10, so he assumed that to find, for example, 5 per cent he should divide by 5. Not all pupil-devised strategies are successful.

Conclusion

When a dyslexic child has difficulty with numeracy, their teacher – and sometimes their parents – may well pick up some warning signs. The next stage is to carry out effective testing and assessment. This needs to cover the three areas explained in this chapter: ability (both verbal and non-verbal), attainment and diagnostics.

Chapter 3
Dyslexia and the Primary Framework for mathematics

The majority of children in primary school follow the Primary Framework. Bearing in mind the difficulties the pupil with dyslexia is likely to bring to the classroom, it is useful to look at just a small section of the NNS guidance, underlining points that are of particular relevance when planning and working with dyslexic learners. The following quotations from the '99 Framework are of particular help when planning and working with dyslexic learners (the italic emphasis is added):

> An ability to calculate mentally lies at the heart of numeracy . . . These skills include:
>
> ○ *remembering number facts and recalling them without hesitation;*
>
> ○ using the facts that are known by heart to figure out new facts; . . .
>
> ○ understanding and using the relationships between the 'four rules' to work out answers and check results . . .
>
> ○ drawing on a repertoire of mental strategies to work out calculations . . . with *some thinking time;*
>
> ○ *solving problems* like [practical, word problems] . . .
>
> In the early years children will use oral methods, . . . moving from *counting objects or fingers one by one* to more sophisticated mental counting strategies. Later they will use a number line or square . . .
>
> . . . and encouraging children to *use this language when they talk about mathematics* is an important stage in developing their calculation strategies and problem-solving skills.
>
> They will develop some of these methods intuitively and some you will teach explicitly. Through a process of regular explanation and discussion . . . *they will begin to acquire a repertoire of mental calculation strategies . . . Not everyone does a mental calculation in the same way (nor is it necessary for them to do so) . . .*
>
> For each operation, *at least one standard written method* should be taught in the later primary years . . .
>
> *Summarising: reviewing during and towards the end of a lesson . . . picking out key points and ideas, making links . . .*

NNS Framework for Teaching Mathematics, Introducing the Framework, pp. 6–8

Advantages in the PNS for the child with dyslexia

Lesson structure

The structure of lessons – with a balance of whole-class teaching and group/individual work, finishing with a plenary – means that the less able pupil benefits both from the mixed-ability approach in which they can learn from their peers and from the opportunity to practise at their own level of ability and attainment. The PNS also allows for work from previous lessons to be reviewed, for new work to be introduced and practised, and for that work to be consolidated before moving on – time permitting.

The PNS recommends that each lesson finishes with a review of the lesson content. Buzan (1990) says that for maximum memory recall we need to review information immediately, at the end of a lesson; then twenty-four hours later; then forty-eight hours later, one week later, and one month later; and regularly every three months after that. Imagine the workload! Nevertheless, the principle of frequent review is well founded.

Doubling and halving

The NNS places emphasis on using doubling and halving for calculations and broad applications. If used correctly, this reduces the number of individual facts that need to be mastered for addition. Doubling introduces the linking of mathematical processes.

> For example, $7 + 7 = 14$ so $7 + 8 = 7 + 7 + 1$ or $8 + 8 - 1$ and $6 + 8 = 14$

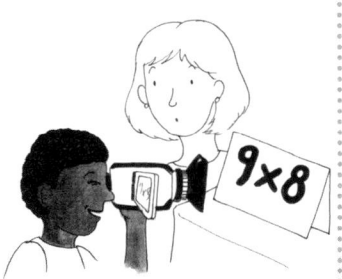

"I'm using a new recording method for this problem."

Halving is harder but equally valid as an approach. It provides a useful tool for division (for example, dividing by 4 can be done by halving twice); and it links to the concept of fractions, where we stress that to find a half we must have two equal parts.

Language variety

The PNS encourages the use of a variety of language and approaches. This offers pupils with dyslexia, and others, the opportunity to hear and use different terms often used for a mathematical operation and to approach a problem in a number of ways.

Linking calculations

The sequential, or inchworm, dyslexic (see page 26) has difficulty in relating and extending mathematical knowledge. Teachers are directed to link various calculations; for example, knowing $20 + 30 = 50$ and $3 + 6 = 9$ means that $23 + 36$ can be calculated.

Recording

The NNS directs teachers to use a variety of methods of recording which allow children with dyslexia to develop their own methods of recording. Care must be taken to ensure that the method chosen is mathematically sound.

Testing

The mastering of procedures and the recall of knowledge can be revealed by the time taken to answer questions. 'Rather than pitch the children against each other, it is better to encourage them to compete against themselves.' This is important for pupils who are processing information slowly.

Difficulties in the PNS for the child with dyslexia

The problems of variety

Although the variety of terms and the understanding of words in a mathematical context must be mastered and alternative methods should be encouraged, there is a danger of muddling the less able dyslexic child by trying to introduce too many alternatives at the same time. Allowing a variety of methods can lead to confusion and to the wrong conclusion.

Memory overload

There is great emphasis in the PNS on mental recall, especially in Reception and Years 1 and 2. The danger for children with dyslexia is that the memory load becomes too great. That often means that there is insufficient time for them to listen, understand and process incoming information.

Input of information

All pupils with dyslexia have to work harder than their peers to achieve the same amount. There are three strands of evidence from research undertaken by geneticists and anatomists into the fast processing of information that indicate that they have problems with the input of sensory information.

'All pupils with dyslexia have to work harder than their peers to achieve the same amount.'

For over a hundred years developmental dyslexia has been thought to have a biological basis. Studies in the 1980s and 1990s confirmed that dyslexia tends to run in families, and various chromosomes have been linked to the difficulty.

The advent of brain-scanning techniques in the 1990s has led to the conclusion that the brain of a dyslexic individual is different from the brain of an individual without dyslexia. Different areas are activated when the two are given two tasks: one involving rhyming, the other short-term memory.

Thirdly, in 1999 research by Stein *et al.* (1999) suggested that individuals with dyslexia have a phonological deficit that is part of a general difficulty in processing rapidly changing stimuli.

As a teacher, it seems to me that because of the difficulty of processing information at speed, the pathways involved – between the various areas of the brain – are likely to become crowded or blocked. This means that dyslexic individuals may well need breaks to clear information presented and to find where to place it before receiving more. Although the PNS allows for time to practise, apply and review what has been taught, the pressure to cover all the relevant objectives can still mean that the pupil with dyslexia does not get the practice and reinforcement that they need.

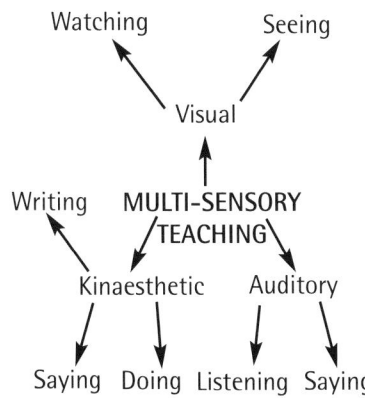

Children with dyslexia need multi-sensory learning and teaching. This means using all three methods of input: auditory (listening and saying), visual (watching and seeing) and kinaesthetic (saying, writing and doing), as illustrated in the figure (left).

Often in children with dyslexia the auditory memory is the weakest. Although concrete materials are encouraged in Reception, during the first two years of schooling the main teaching and learning method is whole class, and auditory.

Initially there was very little in the NNS about using concrete apparatus. It is now increasingly used, not only in Reception and for special needs, but by teachers in general. However, the emphasis is still on discrete pictorial/representational materials – namely number line and square. A variety of concrete materials linked to the NNS and to the PNS are being produced commercially (see table below). These materials should be on the desk for every learner, not just the dyslexic ones, and should not disappear at a particular stage. They should still be available in secondary school. All learners will benefit from the inclusion of concrete apparatus in a lesson. The teacher should use the apparatus at all times, with all learners if possible, when explaining any point. In this way it will become an integral part of every lesson.

'All learners will benefit from the inclusion of concrete apparatus in a lesson.'

Examples of concrete materials
The learning styles of inchworm and grasshopper used in this chart are explained on page 26.

Inchworm	Grasshopper	Both
Pegboard and pegs	Cuisenaire® rods	Numicon®
Drinking straws	Base 10 blocks	Money
Abacus		Unifix® cubes
Geoboards		Wooden numerals
		Dice
		Polyhedra kits
		Decimal sets (Taskmaster)

Rote learning
Be warned! It is possible for a child to 'learn' much of the early number work in the PNS by rote and a stimulus–response reaction. A parrot could be taught to recite number bonds, but it will never understand what they mean. Children may learn that when a teacher asks, for example, 'What is 7 add 2?' the response wanted is '9'. Understanding what is happening is a separate issue. Concrete apparatus is necessary for the less able child to visualise the concepts.

Pupils with dyslexia who have poor memory skills will often rely on memory to learn the procedures necessary for harder multiplications and divisions. The procedure may be incorrectly learned and incorrectly reproduced. It is easy for a teacher to think that a learner has the right idea and just needs more practice, when what is really needed is to go back to the beginning so that the whole process is understood before it is practised and learned.

Questions and answers

Both the first and the plenary parts of a lesson often involve question-and-answer sessions. Pupils with dyslexia often find it difficult to explain their thinking in front of their peers. We need to remember that they need more thinking time too. They are also more likely to panic in a stressful situation, and the knowledge they may have may be harder to locate. Nor is asking a pupil with dyslexia an easier question always the answer. Some children with dyslexia do not have difficulties with the concepts of maths; their problems are with language and/or numeracy. Expecting them to cope at an easier level does not allow them to show their real ability. All too often the child with dyslexia has problems that are not truly defined and as a result they are put with a low-ability group. It may be better to put them with a high-ability group and provide support in reading and/or numeracy. For group work, pairing one of the better readers with a child with dyslexia, who can do the maths but not read the question, provides mutual support. All pupils know when a question is easier and are aware of the competitive nature of the question-and-answer session. If the answer to a question known to be easy cannot be given quickly, then the pupil's confidence and self-esteem are diminished in front of their peers.

'Pupils with dyslexia often find it difficult to explain their thinking in front of their peers.'

The main teaching point

For the main teaching point the NNS says 'tell pupils what work they will do, how long it should take, what, if anything, they need to prepare for the plenary session and how they are to present it; maintain pace and give learners a deadline for completing their work' *(NNS Framework for Teaching Mathematics,* Introducing the Framework, p. 14).

The list of instructions may be too long for the child with dyslexia to remember. Most of us can hold up to about seven items on our short-term memory 'shelf'. Many children with dyslexia have shelves that can only hold three, or perhaps two, items. Ideally, learners should repeat the instructions back. A teaching assistant can help, perhaps making notes about what has to be done. This does not necessarily mean writing down the instructions; it may involve using cartoon pictures or icons – initially agreed with the learner, and later produced by the learner, with help from the teaching assistant – to offer memory support. For example, a simple sketch of a pencil and one matchstick man can mean individual work to be written down. A box with a few arbitrary numbers written in it could indicate use the computer or a calculator.

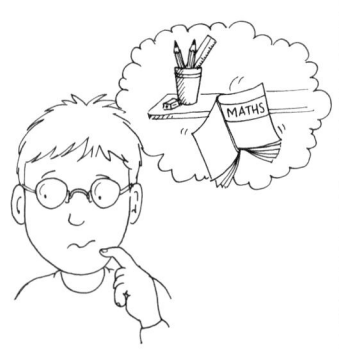

"What subject are we doing?"

Questions that are 'all the same' – for example all addition – may be tackled fairly successfully. Test situations in which the operator may change for each question need practice. This can be one of several reasons why learners who seem to be coping well in the classroom perform less well in SATs and so on. Don't forget that for mental addition we add the 10s first, but for some methods of written addition we teach 'add the units first'. This apparent changing of a rule can be confusing, as can the fact that addition and multiplication can be done either way round (commutative) whereas subtraction and division must be done in standard order.

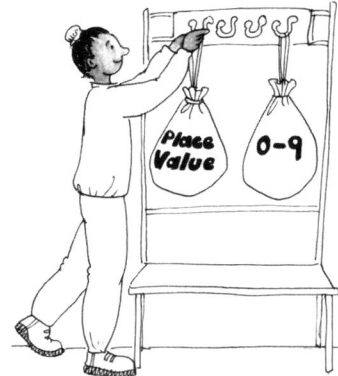

For the majority of learners the PNS's primary reliance on memory, sequencing and number patterns will work well. A few learners will need extra hooks on which to hang their knowledge. Allowing for the fact that some children with dyslexia have strong visuo-spatial skills, it seems sensible for teachers in individual or group sessions to offer pupils who are struggling and may be dyslexic other approaches than finger and recitation. These are explored in Chapter 5.

Conclusion

The Primary Framework for mathematics has many strengths for the child with dyslexia. The latest figures indicate that the aim of 75 per cent of children reaching specific goals by the age of 11 has almost been achieved. However, we must ask where the child with dyslexia will be. The answer in most cases is in the other 25 per cent. Clearly, the NNS has been working for the majority. With appropriate planning and action on the part of teachers and teaching assistants, we can work within and beside the new PNS to the benefit of the child with dyslexia too.

Chapter 4
Focus on mathematics

This chapter will cover:

- ❖ the three components of mathematics;
- ❖ preferred learning styles;
- ❖ the levels of mastery of mathematics.

The three components of mathematics

Let us look at how a child with dyslexia and numeracy skills approaches a maths task. This information is based on work by Professor M. Sharma.

Professor M. Sharma of the Institute of Mathematics, Massachusetts, USA, has worked extensively with learners who have difficulties in mathematics.

Every topic in mathematics consists of three component areas: language, concept, and numeracy and procedure. Each has to be mastered. A problem in one area will often affect performance in the others. Of the three areas the most difficult to teach, and the most important to master, is concept. Language skills and procedures can be taught. Much of primary-school mathematics may seem to revolve around numeracy, but some compensation strategies can be suggested, especially to older pupils. Without a good understanding of the concepts involved, however, the subject cannot be mastered. A multi-sensory approach, including concrete apparatus and practical examples, must be included in a teaching programme for it to be of lasting benefit to children with dyslexia, as we shall see in Chapter 5. It is worth bearing in mind that what is of benefit to a child with dyslexia will also be of benefit to a non-dyslexic one.

Preferred learning styles

Observations of children learning mathematics have led to the conclusion that they tend to approach and learn mathematics in two ways, first documented by Descartes (1638, cited in Krutetskii, 1976). These were labelled 'grasshopper' and 'inchworm' by Bath *et al.* (1986) and 'qualitative' and 'quantitative' by Sharma (1989, 1990). Current terms include 'holistic' and 'sequential'. The grasshopper and inchworm labels are perhaps the easiest to understand.

Learning styles

The inchworm prefers to learn and follow a formula or recipe, whereas the grasshopper prefers controlled exploration (Bath *et al.* 1986) by taking a question and using learning in a related area to find the answer. The grasshopper approach often means a greater understanding of mathematical concepts and an ability to relate various concepts between different areas of mathematics.

For children with dyslexia who have problems with short-term memory, the learning of procedures is difficult. Those who take the inchworm approach and rely substantially on faulty or poor memory skills will only partially, and often incorrectly, learn the procedures they wish to master.

Inchworm	Grasshopper
Prefers to follow a rule	Controlled exploration
Method driven	Answer driven
Tendency to see topics in isolation	Links concepts and topics
May have poor grasp of concepts	More likely to understand concepts
Does not experiment with solutions; sticks to one method	Will experiment with solutions and alternative methods
Prefers to write everything down	Prefers to work without writing everything down
Tries to remember areas that are not understood and to reproduce procedure by rote – often incorrectly	May have difficulty explaining logic and verbalising solutions
At some stage the reliance on memory will be insufficient (the grasshopper approach is particularly relevant for mental calculation)	Must be aware of inchworm approaches as alternative methods, especially when recording solutions
A calculator should be used with care as it may mask an underlying lack of understanding	May benefit from the use of a calculator to help with basic numeracy so effort can be put into higher-order mathematics
Finds checking solutions difficult and often simply works through the question again in the same way	Has a feel for an answer and can use other methods for checking

For example, consider 29 x 8

Inchworm	Grasshopper	
29	30 x 8	= 240
x 8	240 - 8	= 232
232	29 x 8	= 232
7		

'For those children with dyslexia who have problems with short-term memory, the learning of procedures is difficult.'

Most people when approaching mathematics have both approaches available to them, and can switch according to the demands of the problem. They will choose the method of solution best suited to the problem presented. However, if a teacher relies heavily on one approach and the child relies on another, then some conflict in learning will arise. Reliance on one method is often seen more in secondary-level maths than in primary. The PNS encourages teachers to use a variety of approaches and the National Curriculum requires 'an acceptable method of recording' rather than stipulating 'the acceptable method'.

The PNS guidelines are built on counting, which is an inchworm approach. However, the PNS also stresses the use of previously known relationships and strategies to solve questions, which follows the grasshopper approach. The instruction 'Show all your working' is still familiar to learners, especially older ones who have not benefited from the NNS. Learners are now taught that there may be more than one acceptable method to answer a question. It may be easier to mark work if a set procedure is followed, but that may not indicate understanding. The work may simply show a learner's ability to follow instructions, or to substitute numbers within a given procedure to achieve the correct results.

Within the constraints of the classroom, changing teaching style and offering alternatives, where applicable and possible, may not be easy. Chinn and Ashcroft (1998) suggest teaching a grasshopper approach followed by the inchworm and then a review of both. The PNS encourages this two-pronged approach. However, there is then a danger that weaker learners will fail to understand any procedure correctly, and will become muddled in their thinking. Making the many links that exist all through mathematics is important if learners are to understand the relationships between the various areas and how topics and subject, as a whole, are structured.

'Remember that teaching the pupil with dyslexia means using structured, cumulative and multi-sensory methods.'

Picking up skills

Many pupils without dyslexia will pick up links and alternative solutions, but children with dyslexia have to be taught them. Remember that teaching the pupil with dyslexia means using structured, cumulative and multi-sensory methods. Rather than introducing every topic as new, it should, wherever possible, be linked to existing knowledge. Alternative methods need to be considered, but care must be taken not to introduce them too close together in case the learner muddles them up.

Having worked with pupils with dyslexia for some years, I am beginning to ask to what extent learning style is innate and to what extent it is related to a learner's ability in maths. If you are 'good at maths', you have the confidence to take risks and to experiment when answering questions. You can afford to make mistakes and will learn from them. If you find maths difficult, you will lack the confidence needed to take a risk and will stick to the safe, rule-oriented method. Success or failure will reinforce one approach more than the other, so the learner will tend to prefer one.

'We should teach to the strengths, whilst supporting the weaknesses.'

Too great an emphasis on one learning style can reinforce this preference, but we all need to be able to use the most appropriate method for any particular question or situation. An awareness of the preferred learning approach enables suitable choices to be made for teaching and learning materials, especially for the introduction of a new topic. We should teach to the strengths, whilst supporting the weaknesses.

As an example, I recently supported a teenage boy, Andrew, in Year 10. Andrew is a bright dyslexic student who excels at computing and is always given the responsibility for the lighting in school plays. His reading is fine, his spelling poor. His main interest outside school is his off-road motor bike. His strengths are in visual processing, visual memory and spatial skills. The mainly spoken, auditory presentation in the classroom was not working and he was falling behind and losing confidence.

When he was referred to me, I realised that he needed a visual and kinaesthetic approach. Money became the choice for numeracy, especially simple place value for both whole numbers and decimals. The motor bike became the focus for applying basic skills and making them relevant to Andrew. I learned a great deal about petrol consumption, speed, horse power, braking and so on, applied to bikes. Andrew, in turn, found that maths could be practical, useful and relevant. He could imagine his bike, which helped him considerably when solving problems. The next stage was to generalise those ideas to other areas. Having found that maths was relevant and interesting, Andrew was prepared to try again and take the risks necessary to begin to understand and succeed. It was not the whole answer to his problems, but it was a beginning.

'Children with dyslexia need opportunities to think out loud.'

'If a child cannot learn the way you teach, can you teach the child in the way he learns?' The PNS encourages teachers to listen to learners and give them time to explain their thinking. No longer should 'Explain what you are doing' mean 'What on earth have you done there?' Talking with and by the learner is vital to ensure their understanding at every level. Precise language is necessary. Children with dyslexia need opportunities to think out loud. The teaching assistant is invaluable in this area. They can sit beside the learner, listening to them reading, planning and executing the solution to a question or problem.

An example of how a teaching assistant (TA) can help is given below. It is part of a conversation between the TA and a Year-6 pupil (P), who has been having extra support and is used to the procedure.

TA: Right, can you read the question to me, please?
P: It says 53 times 42.
TA: Do you know what that means?
P: Yes, I have to multiply 42 by 53.
TA: All right. How are you going to start?
P: Can I write it down?
TA: Can you remember what Mrs Grainger said?
P: Um. No.
TA: Do you think you will need to write down your calculations?
P: What's 'calcations'?
TA: The way you work out the answer, showing all the steps you've used.
P: Oh yeah! I need to do that.
TA: Right, so can you write down your calculations as we go through the question?
P: I'll try.
TA: Good, off we go then. Where do we start?
P: Can I draw a diagram?
TA: Of course. Here's your squared paper.

At this point the pupil drew the diagram on the left.

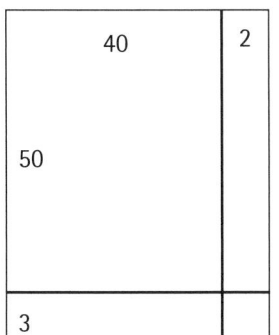

P: Now I can work out the bits and add them together.
TA: Wait a minute. What do you usually do at this stage, before you start with the actual numbers?
P: Don't know.
TA: Just think, wouldn't it help to have an idea of how big the answer should be?
P: Oh yeah! I hestimate, don't I?
TA: Yes, you estimate the answer.
P: I know, I say it's about 50 times 40 which means 5 times 4 and times 10 twice, so we have 20, then two more noughts, which is 20 and nought and nought. *[They wrote 20 and added noughts as they spoke.]* That's two thousands.

The pupil then wrote the following numbers and said them out loud.
I've done 50 times 40, it's two thousands. Now I have 50 times 2, which is 100, that's easy. Um, 40 times 3 is . . . Um . . . Oh, I know, it's 3 times 40, which is 120. That's it. Now I add the answers.

TA: Are you sure? Look carefully. Have you really finished?
P: Yeah, look, I've done that bit, that bit and that bit. Um. I've missed the little bit, haven't I?
TA: Yes, but never mind. Do it now.
P: OK, it's 3 times 2, which is 6. Now can I add?
TA: Yes.
P: It's 120 plus 100, which is 220.
TA: Make a note of that so you do not have to rely on remembering it.
P: OK. Plus 6 which is 226. *[They then wrote that down.]* Now what's left?
TA: Why not cross off those you've already added?
P: Yeah, OK. So I'm left with 2000 to add to 226 which is . . . Um . . .
2, 2, 2, 6.

They then wrote 2226.
TA: Can you read that number to me?
P: Yeah, it's 2000, 200 and 26.
TA: Great, well done! Do you think you're right?
P: Don't know, but it's close to my hestimate, so I suppose so.
TA: Right, let's go on to the next question.

Notice that the TA does not correct the child's mispronunciations but takes the opportunity to use the correct versions herself. She also offers an explanation for a word they do not recognise, and uses it again. The child uses a method that has a high visual content and was originally learned using concrete apparatus. Their confidence when using this method is reasonable, especially when the TA is overseeing. At this stage, when left alone the child tends to panic and make mistakes. They need more practice with this method before trying alternatives.

Allowing pupils to talk is part of multi-sensory learning and enables the teacher to gain some insight into their learning process without extensive testing. More details of this are given in Chapter 5.

Building foundations

The teaching and learning of mathematics is like the building of a wall that takes eleven years to complete. The wall needs firm foundations. Without those foundations it will become unstable. Cracks will appear and it may even fall down, either in part or as a whole. The foundations may be covered over so that cracks are seen in the wall itself and not necessarily in the foundations. Papering over these cracks, or filling them with filler, will not cure the problems. The cracks will reappear and may get bigger. What needs to be done is to reinforce the weak foundations. Extra support teaching has to return to the beginning, and treat the underlying difficulty rather than the symptoms.

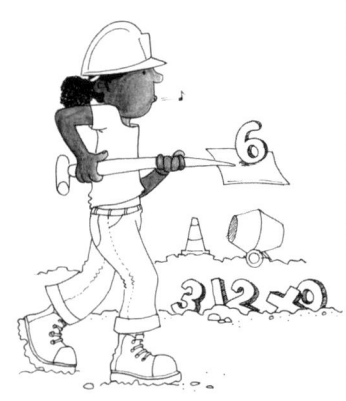

"I'm building my mathematical foundations."

For example, the child who cannot understand decimals may never have understood place value with whole numbers. They may have been able to cope with whole numbers by relying on memory and knowing that following a particular procedure produced an answer that received a tick from the teacher. This strategy cannot be extended when faced with decimals. Understanding is needed to extend concepts – memory alone is not sufficient.

Just as we need the correct tools to build the wall, we need the correct tools to teach and learn mathematics.

The PNS provides the classroom teacher with a detailed guide for teaching numeracy. As teachers, we must be aware of what a topic or task involves mathematically, and how it relates to other topics.

For example, how does an algebraic equation of the form $2 + 4x = 18$ relate to $2 + 4 x 4 = 18$? Problems with decimals often relate to basic difficulty with place value for whole numbers, which are mastered more by rote than by understanding.

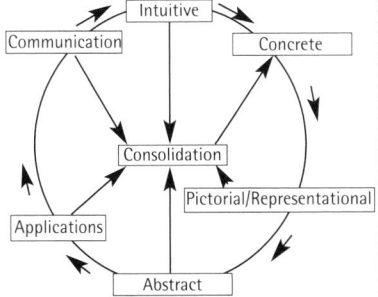

This task analysis is central to the planning of teaching programmes, both in the classroom and for individuals. Controversy exists about the validity of various philosophies and approaches (Daniels and Anghileri 1995). However a structured hierarchy, such as the one in the diagram in the margin, can at best provide a structure to follow, and should at least offer the teacher a way to understand how mathematics is learned.

Levels in the learning of mathematics

Levels in learning do not relate to the subject hierarchy (the mathematical wall). They relate to the way the brain responds to incoming information and the order in which it should be introduced so it can be dealt with efficiently. In mathematics in particular there is a very clear hierarchy of learning. Ideally, teaching should follow this.

Much of higher-level mathematics is taught at the abstract level and it is increasingly possible, especially with the use of computer graphics, to illustrate the theory. The diagram on the left adapted from that proposed by Sharma (1990) shows clearly the levels that need to be mastered in the learning of mathematics, and their order. They are clear, easily understood by a teacher, and they have been found to be effective in the teaching of children with dyslexia. Sharma proposes starting with the intuitive level and moving clockwise. At all levels consolidation is imperative.

The diagram suggests how work can be presented and learned. Wherever one begins in the hierarchy, it is possible to move to another stage, always remaining aware of the need to consolidate.

Let us take a look at the levels in detail:

- ❍ Intuitive: At the intuitive level material is connected to something that is already known. For example, a child learning percentages may, and should, connect them with both decimals and fractions. This connection is not made because the teacher explains it. It is made when the learner makes the connection for themselves. However, errors of connection may be made. For example, I once taught a child with dyslexia who always sat in the same place when I was with her. She decided she had to sit at a particular table when practising multiplication tables.

- ❍ Concrete: At the concrete level apparatus or materials are needed to practise and reinforce rules, concepts and ideas. This level should be used both in its own right and, whenever possible, to provide tactile and kinaesthetic experience to reinforce all levels.

- ❍ Pictorial/Representational: At this level a picture or diagram is needed to solve a problem or prove a theorem. Like the concrete, this level should be used both in its own right and, whenever possible, to provide reinforcement. It is more obviously included for some areas of mathematics such as geometry, trigonometry and statistics.

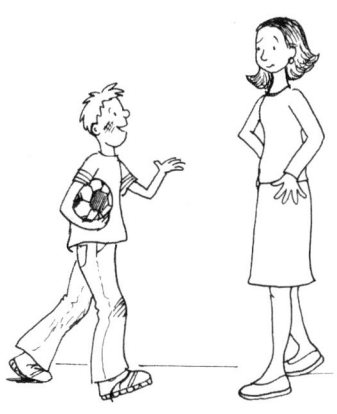

"I've been reviewing my shape and space knowledge."

- **○** Abstract: At this level the child can deal with symbols and formulae. Sharma suggests that it must be reached to succeed in examinations. When mathematics is introduced at this level, many pupils with dyslexia will find it hard to understand.

- **○** Applications: At this level a previously learned concept can be applied to another area or subject. The grasshopper will find this level easier than the inchworm.

- **○** Communication: This is the highest level of learning. To convey our knowledge to others is a reflection of true understanding.

For the child with dyslexia we must add, at all levels, the level of consolidation. Once a topic has been taught and understood it cannot be assumed that it will be completely assimilated. An ongoing process of review must follow everything taught and learned. This may, at some levels and for some topics, be partially undertaken by playing a game and/or using the computer. For example, the computer program NumberShark (from WhiteSpace) offers a wide variety of activities, which give opportunities to practise topics in an enjoyable way (age range 7–14).

Remember that none of the above levels will stand alone. Each must fit and link with the others. We shall now focus on one that impacts on all the others.

Concrete

Concrete materials should be available to all learners so that all can benefit and the dyslexic child will not feel singled out. The teacher must not dictate when they should be abandoned; it must be the decision of the pupil to forgo their use. If a learner wants concrete aids to help with questions, their use should be continued. The pupil is usually the best judge of their own capability.

It is vital that learners work from the concrete through to the representational and abstract. Initially learners work orally when using concrete apparatus. They then progress to having a teacher or TA recording what is being done (using numbers). Then the learner, whilst still using the apparatus, does their own recording and finally records without the need of the apparatus. This can be effected using boxes. The method is shown on the left.

An alternative is to use a tens and ones sheet, as illustrated on page 33. This sheet should be laid on a table, the materials (e.g. rods) placed on it as shown. Initially the pupil works on the paper, saying out loud what they are doing. Then the process can be repeated, with a TA recording. The next step is for the pupil to use the materials and to record themselves. Finally they record without using the materials.

Tens and units: concrete to symbolic

Materials:

Two open boxes
Cards (two sets) with digits 0 to 9
Cards (two sets) with digits 10 to 90
Drinking straws or 'tens and ones' rods
Sheets ruled up with tens/units columns

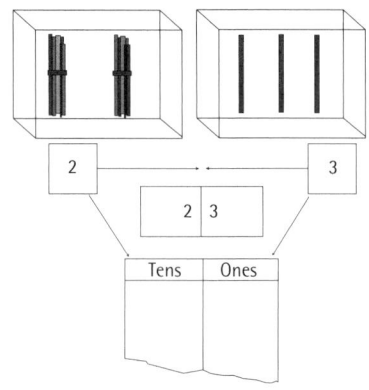

Example: 21+17

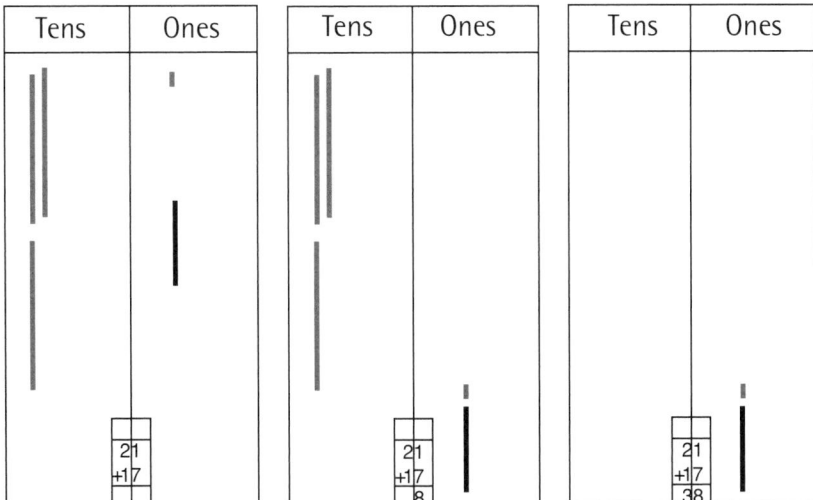

Sometimes pupils need the concrete apparatus as a confidence prop. Great encouragement may be needed for it to be abandoned.

Returning to the analogy of the wall, each part, or brick, is joined to another.

'Mathematics should not be seen as a collection of isolated facts and concepts.'

Mathematics should not be seen as a collection of isolated facts and concepts, as is often the view of the dyslexic inchworm. The more connections that can be made in mathematics, the lighter the memory load and the easier it is to see the inherent logic. Algebra is not separate from arithmetic. Mathematics is like a tree. The roots are the pre-skills needed for mathematics, and the trunk is the numeracy out of which come the branches that grow into areas such as algebra, geometry, trigonometry and, later, calculus.

Much of mathematics, certainly up to GCSE level, is taught 'bottom up'. It starts with particular, simple examples, which may at primary level be illustrated with apparatus, and may at secondary level begin at the pictorial level. However, most A-level mathematics, particularly in the areas known as pure maths, is taught 'top down', from an abstract level.

A small percentage of learners, who may even have achieved an A grade at GCSE maths, suddenly find that the A-level approach does not fit their way of thinking. These students will often struggle and may give up the subject altogether. Some have their confidence shattered and feel that they are letting themselves and others – parents and teachers – down. Unfortunately some receive little sympathy and understanding from adults, who may assume that, because the learners did well at GCSE, they should have few problems with A-level. If learners understand their own learning style (metacognition) and know their own strengths and weaknesses, that will not necessarily make the problems go away, but it will help to boost their confidence and self-esteem, which we all need to succeed at any given task.

Solving a dilemma

Let us return to the processing of information, which we have seen is accepted as being slower for children with dyslexia, and to short-term/working memory, which is often poor. In the classroom this often means that the child with dyslexia gets left behind. While they are still struggling to familiarise themselves with one procedure or topic, the rest of the class is ready to move on. This poses a problem: if a topic is left so that the next one can be followed, it will not be learned, understood correctly or reinforced sufficiently. However, if the learner perseveres at their current position, they will miss the vital information being given or discussed for the next topic. Keeping a child in to complete work or to gain more practice may seem to be a solution, but it is associated, by both learners and parents, with punishment and failure. How can we maintain the child's confidence and provide adequate learning time without depriving them of other activities?

The computer can play a major part in this situation. The learner can be encouraged to use selected programs to practise and reinforce teaching points in an enjoyable way. At a basic level, where many of the problems start, parents can also help by playing both board and card games, most of which involve at the least an element of counting.

I, and most of my colleagues, also use maths cards, examples of which are shown in the photocopiable resources. We also use precision teaching (see page 51) and give the children activities to be completed at home. However, it must be stressed that these need to be used with care, taking only a few minutes to complete and with the agreement of the learner.

Conclusion

In this chapter we have found that before thinking in specific terms about the teaching and learning of mathematics, we have to be aware that in mathematics there are three components, preferred learning style and levels of learning, all of which we need to consider.

There is a danger that the emphasis on numeracy in the PNS may make us fail to see where we are eventually going, or hope to go, when we teach our children. We need to be aware of differing learning styles, but should not place too much emphasis on them. Although the PNS guidelines encourage teachers to teach a variety of approaches, we must take care not to muddle the weaker learner. Equally, too much emphasis on one method may stop the weaker learner from using the approach that they prefer. For us as teachers, there is a fine line to follow.

Lastly, we need to take on board the levels of teaching and learning proposed by Sharma. They have been shown to help not just the child with dyslexia and others with difficulties in mathematics, but all children who are being taught the subject.

Chapter 5
Strategies for support

This chapter will cover:

◐ considerations when teaching mathematics to the child with dyslexia in the classroom;

◐ ideas for individual support for the child with dyslexia;

◐ the use of a calculator.

'Encouraging a variety of teaching and learning approaches gives learners a choice.'

Encouraging a variety of teaching and learning approaches gives learners a choice. However, it must be appreciated that weaker, less confident learners often want the security they find in being given one method to follow. When presented with a variety, these learners may not be in a position to select the best one for them. They often choose the most structured – the inchworm – process. They then rely on reproducing the method correctly to gain the correct solution, rather than understanding what they are doing. When we remind ourselves of their weaknesses in sequencing and short-term/working memory, it is no surprise that these learners often fail. Failure tends to lead to lower self-esteem and self-confidence, making pupils reluctant to attempt anything further.

Good mathematicians can often answer questions correctly by reproducing a given method and after considerable repetition will gain understanding. The weak learner will try to follow a method but, apart from having difficulty in following the sequence correctly, will also not gain understanding. That comes from hearing, seeing, saying and doing – making maths multi-sensory.

In the NNS lessons vary from about 45 minutes to an hour in length. The first five to ten minutes are spent mainly on practising and reinforcing previous work. The main teaching activity introduces a new teaching point and allows learners to practise, in groups and/or individually. The plenary session is, in essence, a review of the lesson.

Clear guidelines on the use of language mean that learners should make the correct language links (the intuitive level of learning). However, often the new teaching point is introduced using a number square or line and so on. This means that the initial learning level is representational. Starting at a concrete level instead means that learners have the opportunity to do, rather than just to see.

Take the example of introducing fractions. Learners can be divided into groups of 3 and given two cardboard Mars bars, pizzas, cakes and so on and a pair of scissors. Each group is told to share the food equally between them. Teacher-led discussion follows for the whole of the class, about what the learners did and how it could be written down, so that everyone understands what is meant.

More examples will be needed, and eventually learners will be able to give their own examples for a variety of given fractions. These procedures are often followed with special needs learners, but others would benefit from them.

Whilst recognising the need for multi-sensory teaching and learning, we must also ensure that the steps from concrete to representational and written recording are small, rather than giant leaps.

The early years and beyond

Virtually no children with dyslexia will be diagnosed in Reception, and few in Year 1. Research – although not recent, based on the developmental theory of Piaget – has shown that children below the age of 7 have somewhat 'fuzzy' ideas about number and number relations, and about the invariant properties of number: 'Number ideas develop very slowly. They grow from an experience base; that is through physical and social experiences each child moves from an intuitive to a more formal meaning of number' (Inhelder and Piaget 1999).

Counting

Brainerd (1973) suggests that young children naturally use ordinal processes, and that early number work should build on this strength. He advocates a lot of counting. His research indicates that ordinal number concepts and facility with natural numbers develop in children before they gain a real concept of cardinal number. A counting approach is the main basis of the early NNS.

Counting is similar in some ways to reciting the alphabet. However, whereas the alphabet is a list of symbols to which are linked – in an apparently arbitrary fashion – names, the symbols used for counting can be illustrated in a concrete, pictorial or representational way, using objects, fingers and so on. For dyslexic children with sequencing difficulties, remembering the sequence and relating the correct number to its quantity will, at the very least, take longer than for others in the class. Extra work will be needed to relate quantity and number.

Watching children play with bricks and similar objects shows how they use concrete apparatus, building, making patterns, beginning to order and so on. In the classroom, young children need to be given opportunities in early number work to use such apparatus to discover relationships and to generalise. A variety of apparatus is needed so that children do not relate to one set only.

Initially children are taught to count. Each child should have a set of up to ten items (Dienes rods, counters, blocks etc.).

- The teacher (or TA) counts 1 to 5, moving an object each time.
- The children count with the teacher, moving their own set of objects.
- The adult says, for example, '1, 2, 3, 4. We have four counters.' The children need to understand that the last number gives the total of objects.
- The teacher asks the children to count, out loud, and move a particular number of objects without help.

- ◐ The teacher asks how many objects have been counted and moved.
- ◐ To relate them to the digit symbols, the objects can be moved so that they are placed next to the numbers on a number line (linking the concrete to the representational).

Activities such as this must be repeated several, often many, times before moving on.

A pegboard and an abacus can also be used for counting, although for the former relatively good fine motor control is needed. The pegs may be quite small and not easy to manipulate.

Writing numbers

'An important step is for pupils then to write the digits correctly.'

An important step is for pupils then to write the digits correctly. Many younger pupils write them incorrectly, often reversing some. The dyslexic pupil tends to persist in this difficulty.

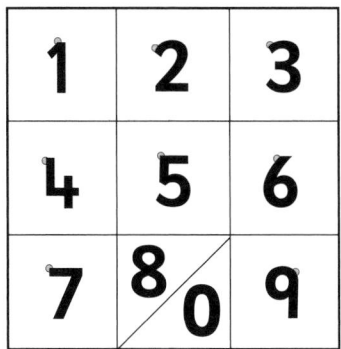

One suggestion to deal with this, using the squared paper that I always use when teaching maths, takes advantage of the fact that the digits from 1 to 7 can all be written to begin in top left-hand corner of a square. Every digit is written in its own square and it must not extend it (see left).

The numbers 0 and 8 are almost impossible to reverse. For younger learners, '9 is naughty 9' and will not do the same as the other digits, so it starts in another corner (the top right).

Note that using squared paper may not work for every pupil. Having tried it with several, I then suggested it to a dyslexic and dyspraxic pupil, aged 8. I'd taken the time to put dots in the right place in preparation for them to write the answers. They came back after a few lessons and announced with glee that they 'had it'. They proved to be writing, correctly if a bit untidily, all the digits the right way round, leaving me feeling quite smug. However, the child brought me down to earth by saying that my method was no good and they had a better one. This they summed up by saying: 'Well, look, 1, 2 and 3 face that way; 4, 5 and 6 face the other; and 7, 8 and 9 go back again.'

Addition facts

When learning addition facts many children want to start at 1 each time. As more and more examples are practised, they become familiar to the child and they develop the ability to start counting on from one number to the next.

For example, take 7 + 4. Going on from 7 we have 8, 9, 10, 11. The child who counts starting from 7 instead of 8 needs more work with the concrete apparatus to see the seven items and then add the four to them.

Here are some examples:

$6 + 3 = 5 + 1 + 3 = 5 + 4 = 9$

$7 + 8 = 5 + 2 + 5 + 3 = 10 + 5 = 15$

'If the child you are helping is having difficulty mastering your preferred method, you need to be able to offer a variety of approaches to help.'

Some children find working with 5 helps with addition and subtraction. Those pupils learn number bonds to 5 and then facts up to 10, such as $6 = 5 + 1$, $7 = 5 + 2$ and so on.

The PNS encourages the use of such strategies, but to many of us who do not have any difficulties with numeracy this use of 5 may seem an unnecessary complication. However, for pupils who are having difficulty, using 5 is an alternative method. If it is also supported by the use of fingers, it can prove valuable. For some teachers, especially those who teach arithmetic without much difficulty and have certain methods with which they are comfortable and confident, the prospect of introducing a different approach can be daunting. Remember that if the child you are helping is having difficulty mastering your preferred method, you need to be able to offer a variety of approaches to help, particularly the weaker pupil.

The PNS stresses that learners should explain their solutions. This can be extended by encouraging learners to explain what a question meant to them and how they worked out the answer. Learners can be encouraged to draw a picture to illustrate the question, or to make the questions into a story. (Questions are commonly used in mathematics – this is known as problem solving – but it is less usual for learners to be given a mathematical sentence and asked to make up the problem.)

With young children I have taken an example like $2 + 3 =$, written it on the board and said something like the example below.

> We have this question. Can you tell me what it says? Good, now we are going to put it into a story. Close your eyes and try to see a picture in your head.
>
> I want you to think about a pond with water in it. On the pond are two ducks. What colour shall we make them? Brown, all right. So, there are two brown ducks swimming on the water. In the middle of the water is a small piece of land, an island. Can you see that? Good! Now, on the island is a small house for ducks. What do you think it will look like? Keep your eyes closed! Now watch the house carefully. There are some ducks inside. Keep quiet, and perhaps they will come out. Remember, we have two ducks on the pond. Perhaps they are eating, and the others will come to see what there is to eat. Look, here comes one, out of the house and into the water. Did it make a splash? Now another one and another, so how many ducks have come out of the house? That's it - three. Can you count the ducks on the pond altogether and tell me how many there are? That's right, there are five. Now open your eyes and we can write that down as the answer to our question.
>
> Now let's try with some other questions. If I give you a question, would anyone like to tell a story?

The procedure above encourages simple visualisation, which is a necessary skill – especially in the more practical areas such as, later on, engineering and architecture. These are the areas in which pupils with dyslexia tend to be more successful.

'The learning of multiplication facts is often an area of concern.'

Multiplication

The learning of multiplication facts is often an area of concern. Not only is it true that the most efficient mathematicians have an automatic recall of basic number facts, but tables are also important in pattern recognition. Multiplication facts, or tables, should be taught, but teachers must be aware that a pupil's difficulty may not be simply in short-term memory and needing to make more links to learn, it may also be affected by poor self-confidence and low self-esteem. The successful learning and recalling of multiplication tables needs to be reinforced every day.

◗ Year 1: Learners are taught to count in 2s to 20, 10 to 50s, 5s to 20+.

◗ Year 2: They are taught to count in 5s to 30+; recall 2 x up to 2 times 10, and 10 x up to 10 times 10; and recall division for 2 and 10 times tables.

It is vital that x 1 and x 0 are included.

Tables can be introduced, initially by using multiples – that is counting in 2s, 3s and so on and then holding up fingers. For example, 6 x 3 means six fingers and 3, 6, 9, 12, 15, 18. If the child with dyslexia has sequencing difficulties, numbers may be left out or given in the wrong order, so we will get 3, 6, 9, 15, 18, 24 or something similar (12 and 21 are omitted).

'Children with dyslexia need to understand before they can learn.'

The child may fail to see the link between multiples and products. Moreover, teaching of multiplication, including x 1 and x 0, must not be seen solely as continued addition. That implies that numbers increase in size when multiplied. The PNS suggests a reference to a rectangular array, but it will help even more if emphasis is put on multiplication as a rectangle. An inchworm learner seems to prefer using discrete or counting apparatus so a rectangular array assists their approach. A grasshopper works better with continuous apparatus like rods, preferring a more holistic approach, so they will generally prefer to think of a rectangular area.

Some children, especially those who are potentially more able mathematicians, are able to learn number bonds and multiplication tables without initially understanding their application. That is not so for children with dyslexia. They need to understand before they can learn. Learning in isolation will not be successful. Emphasis on multiplication producing a rectangle allows direct links to be made to the finding of an area and to the multiplication of fractions, decimals and percentages and to division. Although the concept of division as the reverse of multiplication is not encountered until Year 3, the foundations can be put in place earlier so that the links can be made when required.

This utilises the intuitive level of learning (see page 31), when we relate new work to previously learned information.

The multiplication tables can be displayed on the classroom wall. They are better presented as individual tables than as a multiplication square. The latter can be problematic for learners with visuo-spatial difficulties. A piece of card

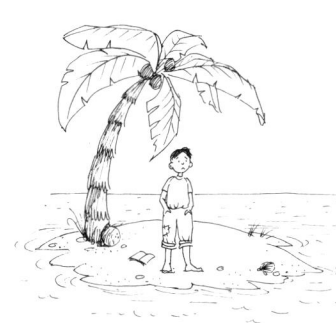

"Learning in isolation will not be successful."

cut as a reverse L is a useful aid to tracking. Every learner can be given their own multiplication card or square for reference. Individual tables are quicker to access, allowing a more immediate response. They show the number patterns and increase the chance of the links being learned.

Further practice can be offered using precision teaching probes (see pages 51) and by the use of the computer. Many computer programs offer practice in multiplication facts in an enjoyable way.

Little and often is what is needed. The teacher must also take the pupil's attitude into account. Some learners, especially older ones, may have so little confidence in their ability to learn their tables that they are not willing to undertake the task. The pressure must be taken off these learners, and support strategies should be offered until they have sufficient confidence in their own ability to try again.

Older primary and secondary learners who are struggling to remember multiplication tables can be taught to produce their own multiplication square. This can be taught to the whole class and is easily mastered if practised regularly. It can be written down in one or two minutes by learners at the beginning of tests and examinations.

The procedure means first reminding children of the commutative property (e.g. 3 x 4 = 4 x 3), so that the square is symmetrical.

The proposed order for teaching multiplication tables and the multiplication square is shown on the left.

The multiplication x 1 need not be included in the multiplication square. The answers for x 10 are easy, so that row and column can be written in. Most children can count in 2s so that row and column can be written down; x 5 and x 9 follow easily.

x 1 (10 facts)

x 10 (9 facts)

x 2 (8 facts)

x 5 (7 facts)

x 9 (6 facts)

x 4 (5 facts)

x 3 (4 facts)

x 6 x 7 x 8 (6 facts)

Don't forget x 0

The PNS puts emphasis on doubling; knowing x 2 will mean that much of x 4 can be added. By using the finger joints x 3 can be worked out. Times 6 is double x 3, x 8 is double x 4 (also for x 8, 5 x 8 = 5 x 9 - 5, 7 x 8 = 7 x 9 - 7, etc.), leaving 7 x 7 as the only one to be learned.

Once the learner wishes to learn, then look for the way that best suits them, taking into account their preferred learning style. Other ideas include the use of tapes, preferably produced by the learner and checked by a teacher, TA or parent, various board games, computer programs and finger tables.

The Egyptian method of multiplication

For example, 37 x 54

	1 x 54 =	54
Double	2 x 54 =	108
Double again	4 x 54 =	216
	8 x 54 =	432
	16 x 54 =	864
Stop here, next number is 64 which is too large	32 x 54 =	1728

$$37 = 32 + 4 + 1$$
$$37 \times 54 = 32 \times 54 + 4 \times 54 + 1 \times 54$$
From above: $= 1728 + 216 + 54 = 1998$

In Year 6, pupils will be introduced to a standard method for long division. This can be confusing for some pupils and using 'guesstimation', as shown below, may be an acceptable alternative. It is based on the principle that division can be seen as continued subtraction.

For example, 6743 ÷ 23:

```
                    23  ⌐6743
       100  x  23 = 2300   2300
                subtract    4443
       100  x  23 = 2300   2300
                subtract    2143
100 is too
big so try 50  x  23 = 1150   1150
                (½ of 2300)
                subtract     993
        40  x  23 = 920    920
                subtract     73
         3  x  23 = 69     69
                subtract      4
Add  293
```

Thus   293 r 4

Finger tables

Sometimes called gypsy tables, these have been around for a very long time. The simplest is for x 9. For this both hands are held up, fingers extended, palms facing the learner. If we want, for example, 4 x 9, we start from the left (some children may need help with left and right) and count to 4. We then bend down the fourth finger. The fingers to the left of this (there are three) give us the number of 10s and those to the right the number of units (there are six), so 4 x 9 is 36 (three 10s and six units).

The finger tables cover multiplication using the numbers from 6 to 10, so they start with 6 x 6, then 7 x 6 and so on. We cannot use any number below 6, but in my experience it is the 6s, 7s and 8s that cause the problems.

We start with the closed fist representing 5, and raise one finger or the thumb (any one will do) on one hand to shows 6, two fingers for 7 and so on. To multiply 8 x 8 you need three fingers raised on each hand. The total number of fingers raised give the tens needed and the number of fingers down in each hand multiplied together give the units; in this example, 2 x 2, which is 4. So, 8 x 8 = 64 (six raised fingers, and two down in each hand multiplied together).

Whether or not a pupil has mastered the multiplication facts, they will by Year 5 have been introduced to standard written methods for multiplication. One method that reflects the emphasis in the PNS on doubling numbers is sometimes known as the Egyptian method of multiplication. It offers a viable alternative to the most common long-multiplication method taught.

Mental maths strategies

As we have said, in the early years of the PNS there is much emphasis on the use of mental arithmetic (or calculation). This is a complex activity involving a variety of skills, in many of which pupils with dyslexia often have difficulties.

Before you read on, write a list of the skills that you think everyone needs for success at mental calculation, for example multi-memory skills.

You should be able to think of such skills as listening, understanding language, concentration, multi-memory tasks, working in competition, working under time pressure, starting/recording the answer, visualisation, logical thinking, number skills, sequencing and watching.

As we can see, the apparently straightforward idea of mental calculation is, in reality, an interaction of a large number of skills. The majority of these skills are areas of concern for most children with dyslexia. We need to recognise these skills and to remember that the PNS says that paper and pencil can support mental calculation. Children with dyslexia will need to use pencil and paper (squared) (see page 45) earlier and more frequently than their peers. It will help them if they can jot down the steps towards solving a question.

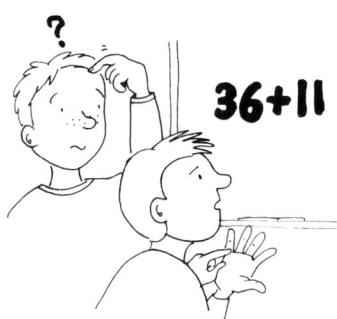

"Mental calculation is trickier than it looks."

'Children with dyslexia will need to use pencil and paper (squared) earlier and more frequently than their peers.'

We must also remember to encourage them, early on, to visualise questions, initially with pictures. Later this can be a matter of visualising the numbers, procedures and so on. An example has already been discussed (see page 38).

Mental calculation has been included in the SATs test, using prerecorded, timed mental calculations. Some learners will struggle because the voice is different from the one they are used to. Most will struggle to keep up with the pace (5, 10 or 15 seconds for a question). This often means that no question is completed successfully and by the end of the test the child is panicking.

A possible solution is for the learner to practise beforehand by listening carefully to the first question and working to complete that, even if the second question is given before they finish. The second question is ignored and the learner waits and attempts the third. Continuing in this way may give the learner the chance to complete half the questions rather than none.

Place value

Some children have difficulty in recognising that size and value are not always related. A variety of apparatus is needed. Initially concrete apparatus relates size to value but learners must move beyond this to learn that position also relates to value. They need to understand that the main reason for this is that we have only ten digits available so we have to have a method for dealing with larger numbers. Pocket wall charts can be used to reinforce the idea that position affects value. These can be made using a large sheet of card on which open envelopes are stuck, as shown in the two examples below. The digits can be written on Post-it notes so they can be easily added and removed.

Pocket chart for addition and subtraction
Example: 17 + 35

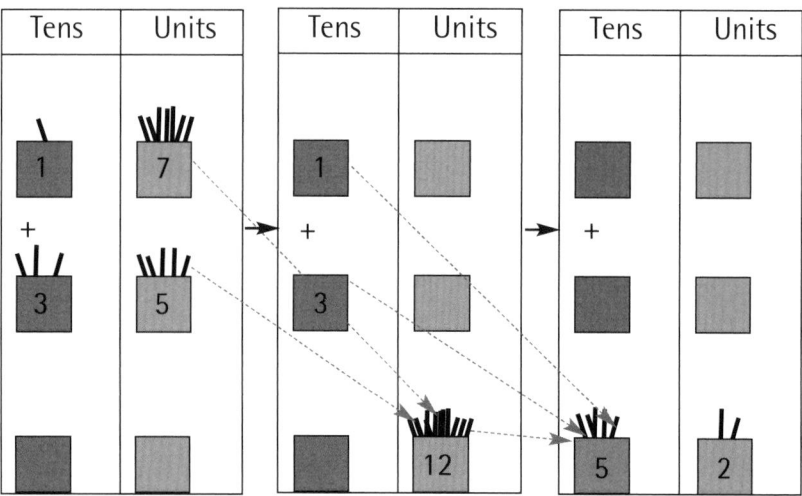

Move the seven and five straws into the 'answer box'.

Exchange ten straws in the units box for one straw in the tens answer box. Move the one and three straws into the tens answer box.

Pocket chart for adding/subtracting decimals
Example: 3.6 + 0.5

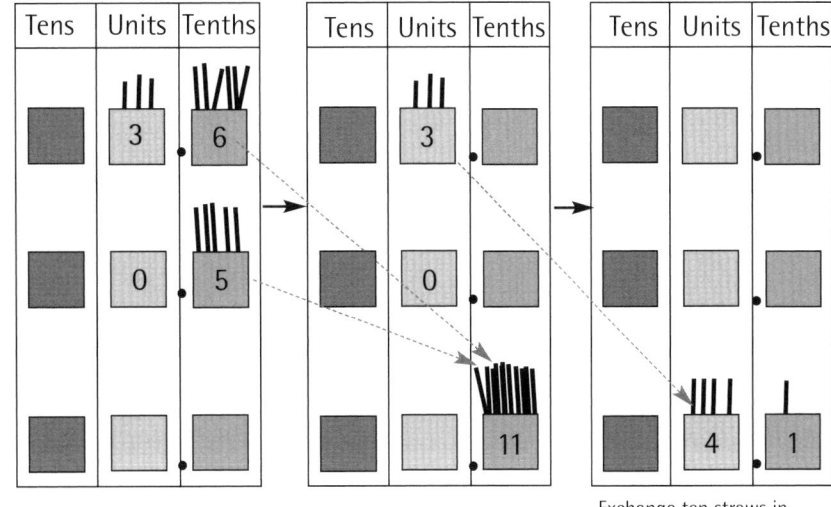

Exchange ten straws in tenths pocket for one in unit pocket.

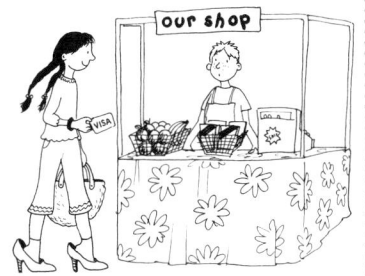

"Young learners are less familiar with money than they used to be."

For older and more able learners money is very useful. It is a practical tool in which size and value are not related. Unfortunately younger learners are less familiar with money than they used to be. The idea of working out how much they have to spend and checking change is becoming a lost skill. Parents can help by taking their children to the sweet shop and encouraging them to decide what they can afford and how much change should be given. Shops can also be a valuable learning resource in Reception and Key Stage 1 classrooms.

Note that the learner who writes teen numbers, in reverse – such as 16 as 61 – may not have a problem with place value. This may be a language problem as we hear the units first but write the tens first.

Linking and extending topics

Directing and promoting the linking and extension of topics in numeracy is actively encouraged in the PNS. This is illustrated by the example of multiplication shown below. Returning to the theme of multiplication meaning a rectangle, which relates to Professor Sharma's approach, we can look at the following diagrams:

For example, 3 x 4:

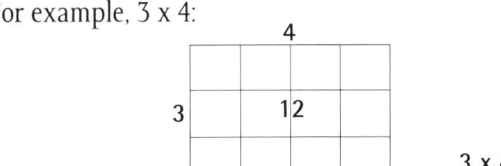

3 x 4 = 12

The diagram illustrates a simple multiplication question and the answer as an area.

Extending this principle to fractions we have, for example, $\frac{1}{2} \times \frac{1}{3}$

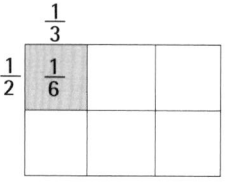

$$\frac{1}{2} \times \frac{1}{3} = \frac{1}{6}$$

This forms the basis for a logical explanation of the multiplication of fractions which does not involve starting from scratch.

Moving on one stage, to decimals, we can also use a diagram, as shown below.

For example, 2.4 x 3.2:

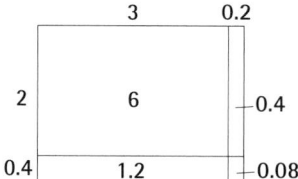

Product = 6 + 1.2 + 0.4 + 0.08 = 7.68

Again, this is not a new concept; it follows on from previous work and can be extended for percentages, as in the example below.

For example, 60 per cent of 200:

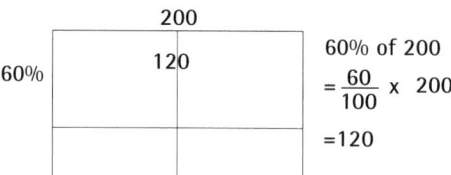

60% of 200

$= \frac{60}{100} \times 200$

$= 120$

Finally, we illustrate the link between multiplication and division and the format used for harder division, not introduced in the PNS until Year 4.

If we return to the first example of 3 x 4 and look at the diagram, we have:

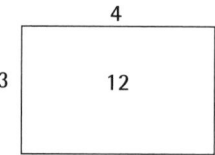

Removing two sides of the rectangle:

4
3	12

Altering the proportions, this can be written as: $3\overline{)12}^{\;4}$

This means that all multiplication involves the same concept and a new concept is not necessary for division, so information is linked.

Note that this illustration can be, and often is, extended further for algebraic quadratic expressions.

A possible approach in the PNS

HEAR – WATCH – DO and SAY

As already pointed out, in the PNS there are three sections in each lesson: whole-class number work, whole-class teaching followed by group and/or individual work, and whole-class plenary session.

This means that any use of concrete apparatus is concentrated in the second section of the lesson, often in the group/individual time.

For whole-class teaching, the child with dyslexia needs work to be presented going from the concrete to the pictorial/representational – not the other way round, as is often done at present. The whole class will benefit from the approach recommended for the child with dyslexia. It means that the new teaching point is introduced with concrete apparatus, used by the teacher, the TA and all children in the class. New work is related to that already known, which will probably be covered in the first section. The introduction is via concrete materials so that children have the opportunity to hear (the teacher), watch (the teacher), do (themselves) and say (think out loud). In this way weaker learning pathways are supported by stronger ones, rather than relying on one way, often auditory, only.

At the end of the lesson all learners would benefit from having individual packs of memory cards (see page 50) to give the extra exposure and practice that many will need.

In the plenary session the work covered is brought together. This is also an opportunity to give learners a very brief overview of what will follow in the next lesson. It gives the less confident learner an element of confidence to be aware of what will be included in the following lesson. If the learner is having extra support, there is an opportunity for discussion about the words that will be reintroduced and new words that will be needed. That helps to avoid the learner feeling that they are sinking because the language is totally unfamiliar to them.

Squared paper
All work done by the learner, and the teacher – whether in an exercise book or a file – should be written on squared paper. This encourages horizontal rows and vertical columns, reducing drifting across the page. (Also, all work should be titled and dated, and if in a file it should have page numbers.)

Worksheets
When worksheets are used to reinforce a teaching point, care is needed to ensure that the dyslexic child thoroughly understands what has to be done. Telling the

child what to do, so that it is not necessary for them to read the instructions, is fine but these instructions may need to be repeated for each question. The child may perform by rote, referring to a previous example for the correct procedure. Children with short-term memory problems will not remember such procedures accurately. They will either be forgotten completely or retained imperfectly.

Worksheets should have the following attributes:
- They should have plenty of space.
- They should be printed.
- They should have a purpose written at the top of each.
- Perhaps they could be printed on pastel-coloured paper. Some pupils with dyslexia find working from black print on white paper difficult because of the contrast. It is easier on the eye to use tinted paper. Some learners ask for very specific colours, and you may have learners with coloured lenses in their glasses. These learners have been tested for scotopic sensitivity and have been found to work better when using these glasses. The learners themselves say that the coloured lenses mean that print remains still, does not swirl and remains in focus.

The use of a worksheet should include talking, which is discussed in Chapter 6. We must remember that many pupils with dyslexia will not finish a worksheet that has been set, which returns us to the dilemma presented earlier. The pupil with dyslexia needs to make more links to learn, so they need more practice, but where do we find the time? Also, they may complete only seven of ten questions on a sheet. Those seven answers may all be correct but result in a mark of 7 out of 10, so to some extent they have failed. This will do little for their confidence and self-esteem. It may lead to a situation where the learner sees little point in trying as they never succeed and they fail to gain that 10 out of 10, which they know they are capable of. Employing the strategies in this chapter and the use of talk will go some way towards helping this problem.

Using a calculator

The PNS recognises that calculators should not be introduced too early in the curriculum. Their primary use should be for checking calculations.

Too early an introduction means that children may fail to make the necessary links or pairings needed for competence in numeracy. Continual exposure and use of number bonds and multiplication tables are vital. Using a calculator reduces this exposure. Most calculators show the answer in isolation, reducing familiarity with sequencing and patterns.

Learners who can recall basic number facts automatically are more efficient problem solvers. Their progress through a question is not diverted by poor retrieval of number facts.

For older learners and adults, a calculator can alleviate the problems of retrieval. It may reduce the chances of forgetting what has to be done to solve a problem when having difficulties with the basic number facts needed to solve it.

There is now a portion of the GCSE examination that has to be attempted without the aid of a calculator. Quite apart from this, there is clearly an argument for discouraging the use of a calculator. One important consideration is the attitude of the learner. If a child, especially an older child, has reached a high level of frustration with themselves when faced with multiplication, adding fractions and so on, the use of a calculator can be encouraged. However, it is as a support tool only, and it must come after understanding. The child must understand fractions or percentages, for example, before you allow them to use a calculator to work them out.

It must be recognised by both the teacher and the learner that some children with dyslexia misread and wrongly write digits and numbers. This is a visual and/or sequential difficulty. For example, 675 may be seen as 975; and 2078 may be entered, or read, as 2708. A calculator that allows scrolling back over previous lines of entry can provide some additional support.

Using a calculator is similar to giving pupils with dyslexia an electronic spelling aid. That does not mean that phonics and the rules of spelling are not taught. It provides an alternative that recognises that the pupil with dyslexia will still have problems with spelling, especially when working under pressure. A calculator should be viewed in the same way.

Helping pupils with dyslexia in the classroom

The chart on page 48 summarises ways of helping dyslexic pupils with numeracy problems in the classroom. It offers advice for early years, primary and secondary pupils. T refers to the teacher and TA to the teaching assistant.

Conclusion

The PNS has many strengths and it offers opportunities for our pupils with dyslexia to succeed. The main difficulties will be caused by memory overload, slow speed of information processing and the pace of the programme. A way needs to be found for learners to have extra time to practise and master procedures.

'Being dyslexic and having difficulties in numeracy does not always equate with low ability.'

We must remember that being dyslexic and having difficulties in numeracy does not always equate with low ability. Many of our children have a good grasp of the concepts involved in maths and can often develop efficient strategies for themselves. We must be careful not to restrict their development in maths because of their difficulties in numeracy.

T	Give instructions in the order they are to be carried out. Poor short-term memory means that more than two or three instructions cannot be remembered by a pupil with dyslexia.
T/TA	Encouraging learners to record working earlier will reduce the danger of overloading their short-term and working memory so they lose their way through a question.
T/TA	Offering learners the opportunity to think out loud is also vital. This gives the opportunity to: ❍ listen to the learner; ❍ understand how they are thinking; ❍ know whether they can access the correct language. A learner who is a very strong holistic thinker may not think in language. A dyslexic sequential thinker may not have mastered the skills and procedures sufficiently to solve a problem. Both may have difficulty in accessing the correct language.
T/TA	Very young children need to be encouraged to visualise questions. Turn questions into mathematical stories (see page 38). Initially, you can make up some stories, but it is vital that learners develop this skill for themselves.
T/TA	Even young children need to be taught and to practise study skills. This includes question analysis and problem-solving techniques (see Pupil support record sheet in Photocopiable resources).
T/TA	Not only do pupils with dyslexia have difficulty in telling the time; many of them are not aware of the passing of time. Younger learners will be helped by seeing a sand timer (these are available for a variety of times) so they can watch time passing though the glass.
T/TA	Children should be given practice in approaching tests and exams, and offered strategies for coping with timed questions in SATs. It is better for the learner to do two or three questions successfully than to get left behind on the first question. That may mean they panic and achieve nothing. Perhaps we need to teach them to miss out alternate questions.
T/TA	Pupils with dyslexia will need to use pencil and paper sooner and more often than their peers.
T/TA	Use squared paper when working with pupils with dyslexia.
T/TA	Always try to sit the pupils with dyslexia where you can see clearly what they are doing. They are more likely than other learners to go off on the wrong track, and they need to be corrected as soon as possible.
TA	Encourage pupils with dyslexia who have a question and cannot ask the teacher immediately to make a note of the problem – they are likely to forget what they need to ask.
TA	When learners are given a list of instructions ensure that the pupil with dyslexia knows what has to be done. The instructions may need to be separated into smaller groups if there are many. However, this technique will not be sufficient by itself; dyslexic learners will need constant reminders to complete all the instructions as they progress through a task.
TA	You can provide a second pair of hands and eyes. For example, if the learner has difficulty separating 3 and 5, + and x etc., then listen carefully to ensure the child names and writes each one correctly. Initially you may have to read or write the symbol for the learner.
TA	Pupils with dyslexia cannot multi-task easily. When working with them, work must be prioritised. If you are working on addition alone, that is a single task; however, when problem solving more skills are involved and they may lose track of what they are doing. Encouraging a learner to think out loud means that you can jot down useful information, and even in some cases provide the answer to the arithmetic so that the learner can concentrate on the problem solving.
T/TA	Concrete materials should be available on every table in the classroom, not just for learners with special needs. This means they are not 'special', and they can be used by you and by learners as an integral part of the lesson – they are there for reinforcement and for added and alternative explanations.

Chapter Six
Making maths multi-sensory

This chapter will look further at:

- the importance of talking and doing;

- the use of memory and key cards;

- precision teaching;

- talking and doing.

The importance of making maths multi-sensory has already been emphasised. Part of this approach involves talking. All teaching of mathematics, especially to children with dyslexia, must contain a large element of discussion. The PNS encourages this approach. It is vital that the child is given every opportunity to talk about the topic and to think out loud. Talking also:

- allows the teacher to listen and hear whether the learner understands what they are doing;

- allows the teacher to hear whether the learner has the necessary language skills to explain what they are doing and whether they can express their mathematical approach verbally (sometimes difficult for the grasshopper);

- makes the learner search for language;

- makes the learner think ahead logically.

Teachers, or a TA, should ask a child to talk through questions and solutions as they work, initially whilst using concrete materials. Every application should have its own, specific, repeated procedure.

One example of this is given below. Anna, a Year-4 pupil, was learning exchange for subtraction. (The NNS uses the term 'decomposition'.) Anna has been asked to find 63 - 39. She has been given a selection of tens and units rods. Her thinking, out loud, was as follows:

> I need 63 so I want 6 tens and 3 ones. *[She took out the rods she wanted.]*
> Now I need to take the nine away but three is not enough and I can't get to
> it. I will have to use one of the tens as I can get nine out of there. So I will
> exchange a ten for ten ones and move them to the ones. *[Whilst talking, Anna
> picked up a tens rod, exchanged it for 10 unit rods and put them with the group
> of 3 units.]* Now I can take the nine away. *[Anna had to check back to the
> question to remind herself what she had to do. She then took the nine away
> from the 10 ones she'd exchanged.]* Um! Now I have one and three – that's 4
> ones. If I take the 3 tens away I have 2 tens left, so the answer is 24. *[She was
> moving the rods around while talking.]*

At this stage Anna is not recording her work symbolically. She has placed the rods on a sheet of paper showing the tens and units columns (see page 33).

'It is the responsibility of the specialist teacher, in particular, to take into account the learner's learning and thinking style and to use it as a strength.'

```
19   8 x 9 = 72, write down 2 and
x8   carry 7
152  8 x 1 = 8, 8 + 7 = 15
 7
```

Using concrete materials, verbalising and writing down is a multi-sensory approach. Having to sequence a question correctly, using the correct language, is vital for the learner. It will also assist the teacher to know whether the child truly understands the task.

Talking through a problem may be especially difficult for the visual thinker. As discussed earlier, much of the mathematics taught in school – particularly in secondary education – may be taught with a sequential, procedural approach; and it is expected that it will be learned and reproduced in a similar way. It is the responsibility of the specialist teacher, in particular, to take into account the learner's learning and thinking style and to use it as a strength whilst improving the weaker areas of language and sequential thinking.

For example, the learner who sees 19 x 8 as 20 x 8 - 8 can be encouraged to use this method for explaining multiplication and checking an answer done by the standard inchworm procedure, as shown on the left.

Finally, it must be remembered that some children with dyslexia will find it particularly embarrassing if put on the spot in front of their peers and asked to explain their thinking. They may have difficulty with word retrieval, which affects fluent speech, and/or lack confidence in their own ability. Such situations need a sympathetic approach. It may be necessary to allow these learners to explain their thinking in an individual, one-to-one situation with a teacher or TA instead.

Memory and key cards

Many of the children will have short-term memory problems. To help children retain what has been taught and learned the key facts can be written on cards. These may be simple symbol cards, with +, x and so on displayed on one side. The words (language) known for the symbols by the child at that stage are written on the other side (see Photocopiable resources for examples you can use). Later we can make key cards showing a rule or formula and a specimen example – for example Pythagoras' theorem. Memory cards, in particular, can be reviewed every lesson, or as needed, to help children retain the information.

An example of a memory card.

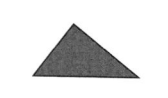

Front

Triangle

Back

The pupil can be shown the front (or can look at it by themselves) and be asked to name the shape. They could also be asked to read the word on the back and/or draw the shape.

The key cards can be used:

- ○ for reference in the classroom (see page 45), as a reminder when working on a particular topic;
- ○ for homework, as a quick learning tool to practise linking pictures, symbols, number bonds etc.;
- ○ when revising, to jog the memory;
- ○ when building on known topics for further work.

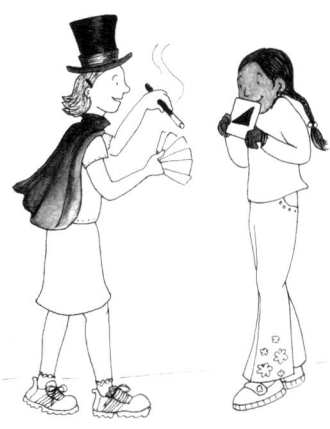

"Your card is a triangle."

Sutton Dyslexia Association produces a useful pack of memory cards.

Precision teaching

Precision teaching is the basis of programmes such as Kumon Maths. It provides repeated practice until a preset standard is reached. It is useful for practising basic number facts, but must be used with care for a child with dyslexia. The inchworm often enjoys completing the probe sheets (worksheets), but may do so without linking any of the methods employed so each probe task is seen in isolation. The grasshopper will often find the repetition boring and deem it unnecessary. If used selectively, precision teaching can supplement or provide an alternative to memory cards.

Precision teaching is a drill and practice method to reinforce basic skills in literacy and numeracy. It can also be used in the following ways:

- learning formulae;
- reinforcing and learning number bonds and multiplication tables.

Outline
The learner is presented with a probe sheet (a worksheet with 100 questions to be answered, words to be read etc.). This is attempted daily, usually for one or two minutes, until the learner achieves a previously agreed target. The success rate is written on a graph. The target level is then raised or, if the rate is acceptable, the probe sheet is presented to the learner at increasing time intervals to boost their memory.

A probe usually follows one of the following:

- see/write (e.g. number bonds), which a learner can do alone;
- see/say (e.g. word reading); which needs input from a teacher or TA;
- hear/write (e.g. spelling), which can be undertaken using a tape recorder.

Detailed procedure
The procedure is as follows:

- Clearly define the task; e.g. number bonds to 10, multiplication by 6.
- Decide on the presentation of the probe; e.g. horizontal addition.
- Write the probe and produce several copies (one probe is used for each task, so it will be reproduced five to seven times for a week's reinforcement)
- Set the expected success level, deciding how much time should be spent on each probe. This can be based on:
  - the pupil's previous success in a similar task;
  - the success of the pupil's peer group in a similar task;
  - asking the learner to attempt the first probe, after which the teacher and learner discuss the result and reach agreement on the required success level. Never exceed a maximum of five minutes.
- Ensure that the learner has been taught the specific skill; e.g. they understand number bonds to 10 and have done plenty of concrete examples.

- Explain clearly to the learner the purpose of the probe and what is involved (the learner must be willing to participate).
- Give the probe to the child to do the first one while the teacher is present, and chart the result. The pupil can work across each row or down each column, but must be consistent.
- The pupil should always read the question and say the answer out loud.
- Explain to the parent what is involved and what the probe is for. For most probes other than mathematical ones a parent will need to be involved.
- Try to present the probe to the pupil at the same time each day.
- The learner should be encouraged to complete the graph themselves or the parent can do this. If not, the completed probes can be returned to the teacher or the TA for marking and charting.

Charting the results

The type of graph paper used is often linear-exponential, which shows rapid improvement at lower levels to provide motivation; but ordinary linear graph paper can be used. The method is as follows:

- Add up correct and incorrect responses separately.
- Mark the number of correct responses on the graph with + and the number of incorrect responses with x.
- Join adjacent crosses with a straight line. Use different colours for correct and incorrect totals. If a day, or days, are missed leave a gap.
- The chart shows the pupil's progress. The number of correct responses should go up to the expected success level and the number of incorrect responses should decline to zero.
- Once the target has been achieved for three successive probes, the task can be considered to have been mastered at that level. Either increase the target level, if applicable, or present the probe at increasing time intervals to reinforce learning.

There are some examples of probe sheets in the photocopiable resources.

Conclusion

If we do not allow learners to talk through their thinking, we do not make maths truly multi-sensory. Everyone learns more from their own voice than from anyone else's – something that we as teachers should bear in mind.

Memory and key cards provide valuable support for all learners, not just those who are dyslexic. They could be used by the class as a whole.

'If we do not allow learners to talk through their thinking, we do not make maths truly multi-sensory.'

Chapter 7
Final thoughts

Most of us cannot imagine what it is like to be dyslexic, but we can all become more aware of the difficulties our pupils with dyslexia often experience with the maths curriculum. Raised awareness will equip us to work sympathetically with our pupils and to provide them with suitable support. What works with a pupil with dyslexia also works with the non-dyslexic. Unfortunately the opposite is not always true.

The theme of this book is to encourage making maths multi-sensory. The PNS goes some way along that route by encouraging children to talk about methods and solutions. It does not, however, make maths multi-sensory in the way that is understood by the specialist teacher. I hope that I have alerted you to the need to use concrete materials as a method of introduction, rather than as an illustration after the use of number lines, squares and so on. Remember that materials alone are not sufficient; they must be linked to the symbols we use for recording mathematical information. Everyone can be given the opportunity to use the materials – not just the weaker pupil in primary school, but pupils in secondary schools also. If it is the norm, it will be accepted by all.

'There is no such person as a typical dyslexic learner.'

There is no such person as a typical dyslexic learner, so we need to adapt our teaching and provide a variety of materials to enable learners to generalise concepts. The materials suggested in this book are just a few of many possibilities.

Most pupils find that apparatus helps understanding. In fact several of the teachers I have trained to teach or support dyslexic pupils in maths have commented that the use of concrete materials has suddenly made clear to them something about which they were not sure.

No book can cover everything teachers need to know about dyslexia and maths; nor should it. You will find out much more about how to recognise and help pupils affected from your everyday experience of working with them.

I hope that you have found this book both useful and informative. At the least, I hope it reinforces the things you already do to support your pupils with dyslexia; and, at the most, that it gets you started and sets you thinking of further ways in which they can be helped.

Just remember: *Make maths multi-sensory for all.*

How parents can help

Teachers are expected to teach; parents are not. Many parents want to help their children with school work, but when it comes to maths they may lack confidence in their own ability, let alone their ability to help others. It is almost acceptable to find maths difficult. Comments I have heard from parents include the following:

- I could never do maths at school.
- I tell him to ask his father/mother/brother etc.
- They use different methods nowadays.
- I can do arithmetic but I can't help now she's at secondary school.

Perhaps the most telling of all is 'I cannot work with my son/daughter; there's too much emotion and we end up rowing.'

One way to involve parents is to have a simple school and home links book which the teacher and TA can use in the following and other ways:

- Write down what has been taught in a lesson.
- Write down homework.
- Explore the use of memory and key cards.
- Explain any precision teaching activities.
- Suggest ways parents can help.

The parent can, in turn, add their own comments, such as the following:

- How the child coped with the homework.
- How long it took.
- If the memory cards were helpful.
- Any concerns they may have.

However, parents can best help their children, especially younger ones, by integrating maths into everyday activities and making maths fun. This does not necessarily mean playing tables tapes on the way to school, although that may be useful. It means trying out some of the ideas in the chart opposite.

We need to remember what happens when children have a skill. For example, those children who can read are more likely to do so for pleasure – children who can spell may play Scrabble®. When you find reading and spelling difficult, you tend to avoid those activities, certainly in games. If a child has a maths problem, they will not want to play maths games.

How parents can help

Reading to a child increases their language awareness, which helps in all areas of education, not just literacy.
Cooking with a child is a valuable activity.
Play a variety of games with your child – not computer games but board and card games. Almost all games involve scoring (usually adding), which children can be encouraged to do. Be careful to ensure that in any game there is an element of luck and enjoyment and that the child has a good chance of winning.
Give your child pocket money to spend in the sweet/paper shop. Encourage them to think whether they have enough money to buy what they want and to check their change.
Give the child a watch that has both an analogue and a digital display.
Do not put pressure on your child. Maths can be fun and useful, which is how it should be in the home.
If you are helping with homework, make sure that the approach you use complements that used at school.
Some children will find it easier to get up earlier in the morning to do homework, rather than doing it in the evening when they are tired. This must be an organised choice, not a last-minute rush.
Suggest that your child plays some computer games that involve logical thinking, rather than just speed of response.

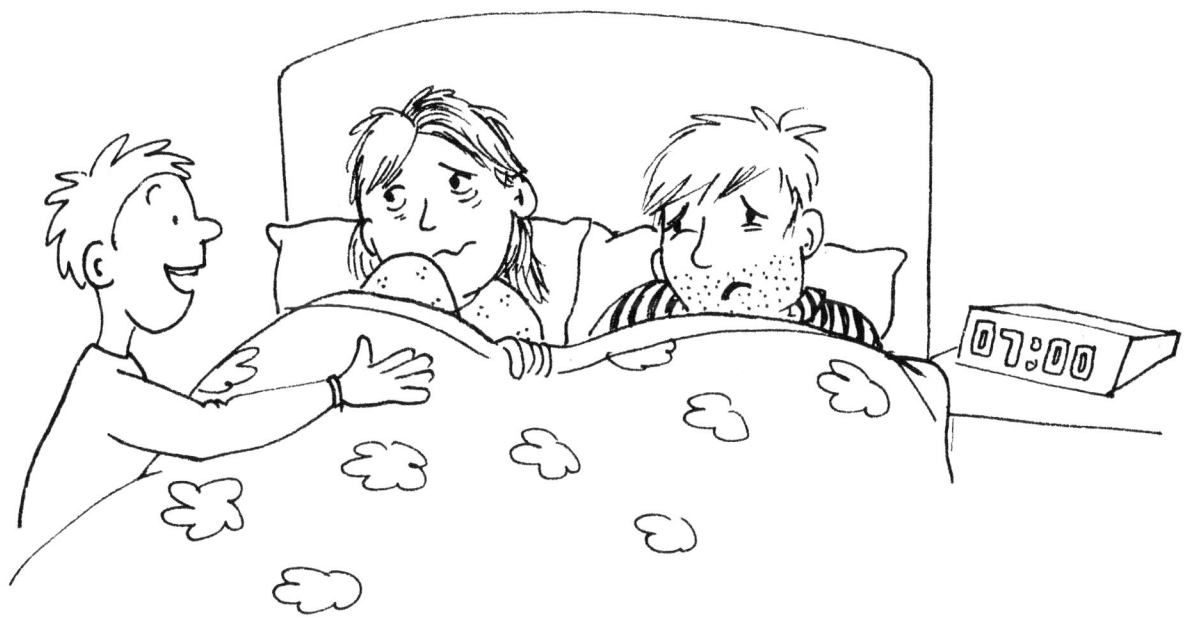

"Are you ready to help me with my homework?"

Pupil support record sheet

Pupil's name .... Class .... Age .... Date of intervention.....................

Symptom	Prerequisite skills	Teacher action	TA action	Time scale	Outcome	Further action
		Teacher's signature	TA's signature			
		Teacher's signature	TA's signature			
		Teacher's signature	TA's signature			

Signed .... Date ....

Thinking about questions

Read the question.

Are there any words you do not understand?

If so, write them in the box and ask your teacher their meaning

Word	Meaning

1. What is the question asking you to find?	2. What are you going to do?
3. What do you need to find the answer?	4. Write down the first expression you need.
5. Make a guess of (estimate) what the answer will be.	6. Now work out the answer.
7. Check your answer against your estimate. Are they close in value? (If not, go back.)	8. Reread the question – do you think you have answered the question correctly?

Memory and key cards

Individual cards can be made with any pupil to practise or reinforce a number procedure or link. Examples are: number bonds, doubling, halving, multiplication facts, language and shapes, definitions, mathematical rules.

These are kept by the pupil and can be run through at home or at any suitable time during the school day. The cards can also be placed on the pupil's desk or table for reference when required. The cards should be small, approximately 5 cm x 7.5 cm.

Examples

FRONT   BACK

4 + 3

3 + 4

7

3 x 4

4 x 3

12

Double 7

2 x 7

14

Memory and key cards

FRONT	BACK

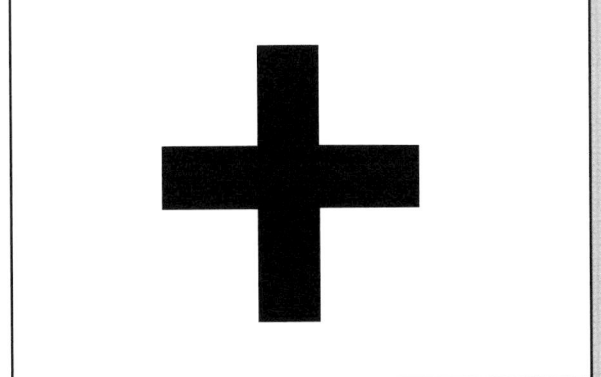

more than
add
plus
sum
total

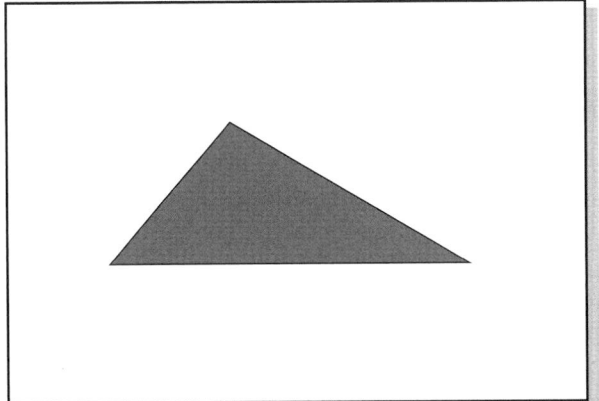

triangle

<u>Dividing fractions</u>
Turn the second
one upside down
and multiply

Example: $\frac{4}{9} \div \frac{1}{3}$

$= \frac{4}{9} \times \frac{3}{1}$

$= \frac{4 \times \cancel{3}^{1}}{\cancel{9}^{3} \times 1}$

$= \frac{4}{3}$ or $1\frac{1}{3}$

---

1 x 2 = 2	1 x 5 = 5
2 x 2 = 4	2 x 5 = 10
3 x 2 = 6	3 x 5 = 15
4 x 2 = 8	4 x 5 = 20
5 x 2 = 10	5 x 5 = 25
6 x 2 = 12	6 x 5 = 30
7 x 2 = 14	7 x 5 = 35
8 x 2 = 16	8 x 5 = 40
9 x 2 = 18	9 x 5 = 45
10 x 2 = 20	10 x 5 = 50

Probe sheet 1

Name .... Date ....
Definition of task: Number bonds to 10 Time allowed: two minutes
Expected success level ....

					✓	✗
1 + 4 =	3 + 2 =	6 + 2 =	5 + 4 =	2 + 2 =		
2 + 7 =	4 + 6 =	7 + 0 =	6 + 3 =	3 + 5 =		
2 + 8 =	3 + 1 =	4 + 4 =	4 + 2 =	9 + 1 =		
6 + 0 =	5 + 5 =	1 + 8 =	2 + 5 =	6 + 4 =		
5 + 2 =	1 + 9 =	3 + 4 =	7 + 2 =	4 + 5 =		
0 + 1 =	2 + 1 =	3 + 3 =	6 + 1 =	1 + 8 =		
5 + 0 =	6 + 3 =	2 + 8 =	3 + 4 =	1 + 1 =		
9 + 1 =	2 + 0 =	8 + 2 =	7 + 0 =	5 + 5 =		
1 + 1 =	7 + 3 =	2 + 5 =	3 + 3 =	1 + 0 =		
8 + 1 =	2 + 7 =	3 + 2 =	6 + 4 =	0 + 3 =		
0 + 0 =	6 + 2 =	4 + 1 =	1 + 5 =	3 + 4 =		
2 + 7 =	4 + 4 =	4 + 0 =	6 + 3 =	2 + 2 =		
0 + 8 =	1 + 3 =	5 + 4 =	4 + 6 =	1 + 7 =		
6 + 3 =	8 + 0 =	4 + 3 =	1 + 1 =	2 + 8 =		
2 + 6 =	0 + 8 =	7 + 3 =	6 + 1 =	9 + 1 =		
2 + 1 =	4 + 4 =	3 + 2 =	2 + 4 =	4 + 6 =		
3 + 7 =	8 + 2 =	3 + 0 =	3 + 3 =	8 + 1 =		
5 + 4 =	3 + 5 =	4 + 1 =	7 + 1 =	3 + 2 =		
2 + 2 =	1 + 6 =	5 + 5 =	9 + 0 =	5 + 4 =		
5 + 3 =	1 + 9 =	6 + 4 =	0 + 0 =	6 + 3 =		

Totals .... / ....

Probe sheet 2

Name .... Date ....
Definition of task: Subtraction to 10 Time allowed: two minutes
Expected success level ....

✓ ✗

					✓	✗
2 - 1 =	3 - 2 =	7 - 5 =	5 - 5 =	6 - 1 =		
9 - 6 =	2 - 0 =	10 - 5 =	4 - 0 =	5 - 4 =		
4 - 2 =	6 - 3 =	0 - 0 =	7 - 7 =	9 - 8 =		
10 - 8 =	8 - 1 =	3 - 0 =	10 - 1 =	6 - 6 =		
7 - 6 =	5 - 3 =	10 - 7 =	10 - 4 =	8 - 3 =		
4 - 0 =	9 - 9 =	8 - 3 =	4 - 1 =	6 - 0 =		
8 - 5 =	10 - 1 =	3 - 1 =	9 - 5 =	7 - 2 =		
7 - 3 =	8 - 7 =	10 - 6 =	3 - 0 =	9 - 8 =		
8 - 4 =	0 - 0 =	8 - 2 =	9 - 3 =	3 - 3 =		
4 - 4 =	5 - 4 =	3 - 3 =	10 - 5 =	7 - 4 =		
6 - 5 =	7 - 3 =	9 - 6 =	5 - 2 =	10 - 3 =		
2 - 2 =	10 - 6 =	6 - 2 =	10 - 8 =	8 - 6 =		
9 - 2 =	8 - 0 =	7 - 3 =	4 - 2 =	10 - 8 =		
7 - 2 =	6 - 6 =	10 - 9 =	4 - 1 =	6 - 5 =		
4 - 3 =	10 - 10 =	5 - 1 =	7 - 2 =	3 - 1 =		
8 - 7 =	10 - 5 =	7 - 7 =	5 - 5 =	9 - 7 =		
6 - 6 =	3 - 3 =	9 - 4 =	10 - 2 =	10 - 5 =		
5 - 3 =	4 - 3 =	10 - 6 =	6 - 3 =	10 - 10 =		
3 - 3 =	8 - 6 =	7 - 1 =	4 - 3 =	8 - 8 =		
5 - 4 =	6 - 4 =	9 - 1 =	10 - 6 =	4 - 4 =		

Totals .... / ....

Probe sheet 3

Name ....   Date ....
Definition of task ....   Time allowed: two minutes
Expected success level ....

					✓	✗

Totals .... / ....

Resources

Suggested reading list

Aubrey C (1999) *A Developmental Approach to Early Numeracy*. Questions Publishing

Baggaley P, Edwards R and Williams A (1993) *Number Activities and Games* (3rd edition). NASEN

Chinn S (2000) *What to Do if You Can't Learn Tables* and *What to Do When You Can't Add or Subtract*. Egon Publishing

Chinn S and Ashcroft J (1998) *Maths for the Dyslexic – A Teaching Handbook* (2nd edition). Whurr

Delaney K, Pinel A and Smith D (2002) *Maths Dictionary*. Questions Publishing

El-Naggar, O (1996) *Specific Learning Difficulties in Mathematics – A Classroom Approach*. NASEN

Gattegno C (1963) *Mathematics with Numbers in Colour*. Available from The Cuisenaire Company, 11 Crown Street, Reading RG1 2TQ

Grauberg E (1997) *Elementary Mathematics and Language Difficulties*. Whurr

Henderson A (1998) *Maths for the Dyslexic – A Practical Approach*. David Fulton

Henderson, A and Miles E (2001) *Basic Topics in Mathematics for Dyslexics*. Whurr

Hillage D (2000) *Count on your Computer*. Available from www.r-e-m.co.uk; lists a wide selection of software to use with pupils with dyslexia, reviewed by the British Dyslexia Association Computer Committee

Miles T R and Miles E (eds.) (1991) *Dyslexia and Mathematics*. Routledge

Yeo D (2002) *Dyslexia, Dyspraxia and Mathematics*. Whurr

Other materials

Amazing Maths (computer program). Cambridgeshire Software House. 01487 741223

Dominoes. Also other ideas for practising time and number. Available from Taskmaster, Morris Road, Leicester, LE2 6BR

Kumon Maths and English. www.kumon.co.uk

Math Magic. Paul Godding, PO Box 260, Newport, South Wales, NP20 4XR

Math Notebooks and videotapes. Mahesh Sharma, Berkshire Mathematics, Chazey Bank, The Warren, Reading, RG4 7TQ

Maths Circus (1–3) (computer programs). 4mation Educational Resources, 63 Boutport Street, Barnstaple, Devon, EX31 1HG. 01271 325253

Memory Cards. Sutton Dyslexia Association, 21 Princes Avenue, Carshalton, Surrey, SM5 4NZ

nferNelson, The Chiswick Centre, 414 Chiswick High Road, London, W4 5TF

NumberShark (computer program). WhiteSpace, 41 Mall Road, London, W6 9DG. 0208 7485927

Stile activities and other materials. LDA, Abbeygate House, East Road, Cambridge, CB1 1DB

Talking calculators. www.rnib.org.uk or www.cobolt.co.uk

Time and Fractions. Xavier Educational Software, School of Psychology, University of Wales, Bangor, Gwynedd, LL57 2AS. 01248 382616

Resources continued

Websites

Basic Skills Agency, www.basic-skills.co.uk
British Dyslexia Association, www.bdadyslexia.org.uk
Dyslexia Action, www.dyslexiaaction.org.uk
Pearson Assessment, www.pearson-uk.com
Hodder & Stoughton, www.hodderheadline.co.uk
iansyst, www.iansyst.co.uk
National Association for Special Educational Needs (NASEN), www.nasen.org.uk
GL assessment, www.gl-assessment.co.uk
The Resource Room, www.resourceroom.net

References

Bath *et al.* (1986) *The Test of Cognitive Style of Mathematics.* Slosson

Brainerd C (1973) 'Mathematical and Behavioural Foundations of Number' *Journal of Genetic Psychology*, 88, pp 221–81

Butterworth B (2003) *Dyscalculia Screener*. nferNelson

Buzan A (1990) *Use Your Head*. BBC Books

Chinn S (2000) *IANS Informal Assessment of Numeracy Skills*. Mark: Markco Publishing

Chinn S and Ashcroft J (1998) *Maths for the Dyslexic – A Teaching Handbook* (2nd edition). Whurr

Daniels and Anghileri (1995) *Secondary Mathematics and Special Educational Needs*. Cassell

Inhelder, B and Piaget, J (1999), *The Early Growth of Logic in the Child: Classification and Seriation*. Routledge

Joffe L (1981) School Mathematics and Dyslexia: Aspects of Inter-relationship. PhD. University of Aston

Krutetskii V in Kilpatric J and Wirszup I (eds) (1976) *The Psychology of Mathematical Abilities in School Children*. University of Chicago Press

Miles T R and Miles E (eds.) (1991) *Dyslexia and Mathematics*. Routledge

Neanon C (2002) *How to Identify and Support Children with Dyslexia*. LDA

Sharma M (1988) 'Levels of Knowing in Mathematics' *Maths Notebook*, 6, pp 1–2. Framingham Ma. Centre for Teaching/Learning of Mathematics

Sharma M (1989) 'Mathematics Learning Personality' *Maths Notebook*, 8, pp 1–2. Framingham Ma. Centre for Teaching/Learning of Mathematics

Sharma M (1990) 'Dyslexia, Dyscalculia, and some Remedial Perspectives for Mathematical Learning Problems' *Maths Notebook*, 7, pp 1–2. Framingham Ma. Centre for Teaching/Learning of Mathematics

Stein J *et al.* (1999) 'Impaired Neuronal Timing in Developmental Dyslexia – the Magnocellular Hypothesis' *Dyslexia*, 5, pp 59–77

Westwood P, Harris-Hughes M, Lucas G, Nolan J. and Scrymgeour K (1974) 'The One-minute Number Test©' *Remedial Education*, 9, 2, pp 70–72

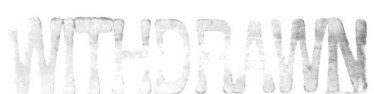

Permission to Photocopy